Y0-AFY-112

Therapeutic Modalities for Athletic Injuries Lab Manual

ATHLETIC TRAINING EDUCATION SERIES

SUSAN FOREMAN SALIBA, PhD, ATC, PT
ETHAN SALIBA, PhD, ATC, PT, SCS
UNIVERSITY OF VIRGINIA, CHARLOTTESVILLE

DAVID H. PERRIN, PhD, ATC
SERIES EDITOR
UNIVERSITY OF VIRGINIA, CHARLOTTESVILLE

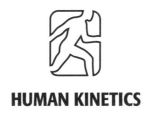

HUMAN KINETICS

Library of Congress Cataloging-in-Publication Data

Saliba, Susan, 1963-
   Therapeutic modalities for athletic injuries lab manual / Susan Saliba, Ethan Saliba.
      p. cm. -- (Athletic training education series)
   Includes bibliographical references.
   ISBN 0-7360-3290-8
   1. Sports injuries--Treatment--Handbooks, manuals, etc. 2. Sports physical
therapy--Handbooks, manuals, etc. I. Saliba, Ethan, 1956- II. Title. III. Series.

RD97 .S35 2001
617.1'027--dc21

                                                              00-066362

ISBN: 0-7360-3290-8

Copyright © 2001 by Susan Saliba and Ethan Saliba

All rights reserved. Except for use in a review, the reproduction or utilization of this work in any form or by any electronic, mechanical, or other means, now known or hereafter invented, including xerography, photocopying, and recording, and in any information storage and retrieval system, is forbidden without the written permission of the publisher.

Acquisitions Editor: Loarn D. Robertson, PhD; **Managing Editor:** Amy Stahl; **Assistant Editors:** Derek Campbell and Susan C. Hagan; **Copyeditor:** Julie Anderson; **Proofreader:** Sarah Wiseman; **Permission Manager:** Dalene Reeder; **Graphic Designer:** Stuart Cartwright; **Graphic Artist:** Denise Lowry; **Photo Manager:** Clark Brooks; **Cover Designer:** Stuart Cartwright; **Photographers (interior):** Tom Roberts (figures 5.3, 12.2, 17.1, and 17.2) and Susan Saliba (all other photos); **Art Manager:** Craig Newsom; **Illustrators:** Argosy (figures 3.1–3.4, 3.6, 9.2, 11.2, 12.1, and 15.1); Tim Shedelbower (figure 9.3, a–c); and Tom Roberts (all other figures) ; **Printer:** United Graphics

Printed in the United States of America   10   9   8   7   6   5   4   3   2   1

Human Kinetics
Web site: www.humankinetics.com

United States: Human Kinetics, P.O. Box 5076, Champaign, IL 61825-5076
800-747-4457
e-mail: humank@hkusa.com

Canada: Human Kinetics, 475 Devonshire Road Unit 100, Windsor, ON N8Y 2L5
800-465-7301 (in Canada only)
e-mail: hkcan@mnsi.net

Europe: Human Kinetics, Units C2/C3 Wira Business Park, West Park Ring Road, Leeds LS16 6EB, United Kingdom
+44 (0) 113 278 1708
e-mail: humank@hkeurope.com

Australia: Human Kinetics, 57A Price Avenue, Lower Mitcham, South Australia 5062
08 8277 1555
e-mail: liahka@senet.com.au

New Zealand: Human Kinetics, P.O. Box 105-231, Auckland Central
09-523-3462
e-mail: hkp@ihug.co.nz

CONTENTS

PREFACE

Skill in modality use requires knowledge of how modalities affect healing and rehabilitation as well as knowledge about when and how to apply physical agents. Certified athletic trainers should be able to evaluate an injury, develop a problem list, and establish treatments that are focused on resolving each problem. Athletic trainers also should be able to document the treatment so that the outcome of the intervention can be determined.

Understanding when and how physical agents should be applied is imperative for the athletic trainer. This lab manual, which accompanies *Therapeutic Modalities for Athletic Injuries,* is designed to provide exercises to reinforce the didactic material presented in the textbook and to give you time to explore the machines commonly used in physical rehabilitation. You also will learn that the principles of a particular modality can be used with many types of machines from various companies. The principles remain constant, and you should be able to use new, similar machines after a brief orientation.

Modality use also has implications for billing and third-party payers, because insurance companies scrutinize the efficacy of modality use. Athletic trainers should be able to justify modality use by developing a treatment plan and should be able to evaluate the continued need for a particular treatment. Additionally, athletic trainers should recognize the limitations of physical agents and should understand that therapeutic exercise is the key to rehabilitation.

Knowing how to apply modalities is a technician's job. Understanding what physical agents can do and at what point in the rehabilitation process they can be advantageous is the goal of a certified athletic trainer.

The laboratory exercises in this manual complement the text *Therapeutic Modalities for Athletic Injuries,* although not all chapters in the text are conducive to lab experiences. These sections of the book should be taught and tested for didactic knowledge but do not have associated psychomotor learning.

LAB 1

General Principles of Modality Use in Athletic Training

Review material from chapter 1, pages 1 to 11 of the textbook, before you complete this lab.

OBJECTIVES

- You will understand that the practice act for athletic training differs by state and that this affects modality use.

- You will understand that reviewing prescriptions and clarifying any discrepancies is imperative before initiating treatment.

- You will be able to identify patient populations that may preclude modality use or require caution such as elderly, diabetic, pregnant, or pediatric athletes.

- You will formulate a systematic method of applying modalities in a safe, consistent manner with a professional demeanor.

- You will understand that the athlete may be apprehensive during modality use and that clear instructions and knowledge of the treatment can dispel apprehension.

LEGAL CONSIDERATIONS OF MODALITY USE

The application of therapeutic modalities often is governed by the medical board of individual states. Many states have licensure for athletic trainers, although a few states do not recognize certified athletic trainers as medical professionals. The Practice Act is the law that specifically determines the restrictions and supervision an athletic trainer must follow. The states that currently have licensure are listed at **www.nata.org.** Because the practice act that governs modality use for athletic trainers may vary from state to state, you should review the laws in your state before using any modality.

Athletic trainers also must follow prescriptions by physicians. Some athletic trainers work closely with a team physician, and often the physician recognizes that the athletic trainer is able to determine which modalities are applicable at certain times during rehabilitation. However, if a physician specifically indicates a treatment, the athletic trainer is obligated to provide that treatment. For example, if a surgeon specifies that active or resistive exercise is contraindicated for 6 weeks after a procedure, then the athletic trainer should teach the athlete exercises that will not compromise the protected structure. Likewise, if a physician requests ultrasound for an athlete, then the athletic trainer should "fill the prescription" or consult with the physician about changes that may be necessary. Merely setting up modalities is a technician's job. It is the athletic trainer's responsibility to understand the mechanism of action of modalities and why modalities are used at certain times, that is, to use modalities as part of a comprehensive rehabilitative program.

The use of modalities involves the application of energy to the body. The energy may be in the form of heat, cold, light, or electricity. Because the application of energy affects various biological systems such as heart rate, blood flow, and blood pressure, you should understand these systems in order to apply modalities safely. Certain patient populations such as elderly, diabetic, pregnant, or pediatric athletes may preclude modality use or require caution. For example, an elderly athlete may have thinner skin, which can burn easily, or may have a significant cardiovascular history or take medication that can affect heart rate or blood pressure. A diabetic athlete may have decreased sensation and poor circulation in the extremities, which affect the feedback necessary to apply electrical stimulation and thermal modalities. No modality should be used on a pregnant woman unless clearly prescribed by a physician, and a pregnant woman's abdomen or low back should never be treated with modalities. Finally, caution should be used with a young athlete because the application of energy, especially ultrasound, may affect growth plates. Always err on the side of caution and ask the patient about his or her medical history.

SYSTEMATIC APPLICATION OF MODALITIES

The following outline presents a systematic method for applying modalities in a safe, consistent manner with a professional demeanor. You should practice these techniques using the step-by-step procedure so you do not forget essential factors. Modifications can be made easily when applying the different modalities.

Applying Modalities
  I. Preparing for treatment
    A. Selecting a modality
      1. Evaluating the injury
        a. Complete a musculoskeletal evaluation of the injury.
        b. Test the temperature of the injured part and make sure the person has sensation in that area.

      c. Determine whether there is edema, noting its viscosity. A softer, less viscous type of swelling is more indicative of the proliferative phase of inflammation. Brawny or thicker, pitting edema is a result of fibrin forming within the exudate or extracellular fluid that has accumulated in the soft-tissue space. Pitting edema leaves a dent in the skin when pressed. The viscosity of the edema helps to determine the stage of inflammation.

      d. Inspect the skin in the treatment area for open lesions, rashes, or scars.

  2. In a clinical setting, check the physician's referral in addition to the evaluation (a physician may request a specific modality treatment).

  3. Establish (or revise) treatment goals. Make a list of short-term and long-term goals. The goals should correlate with a problem list generated from the evaluation.

  4. Select a modality that is best suited to reaching these goals. Keep contraindications in mind.

      a. Evaluate whether the athlete has any additional medical conditions (e.g., diabetes) that may preclude the use of modalities. Use caution with any individual who has a significant cardiovascular history.

B. Checking the machine for safety

  1. Check the condition of the electrical cord. Plug the unit into a ground fault circuit interrupter when a modality is used near water.

  2. Check the temperature of whirlpools, hydrocollators, or paraffin or fluidotherapy units. Turn on the agitator before you check whirlpool temperatures.

  3. Make sure all output intensities of electrical stimulators and ultrasound machines are at zero.

  4. Turn on the power to the machine before connecting the patient, because there is a possibility of a surge when the power turns on.

C. Instructing the athlete

  1. Explain the rationale of the treatment in a way that the athlete can understand.

  2. Explain the procedure so that the athlete knows what sensation to expect. Remind the athlete that hot packs, ultrasound, and many modalities should not be painful, and that the athlete should tell you if these modalities cause pain.

  3. Demonstrate the application if the athlete appears apprehensive.

D. Positioning

  1. Position the athlete comfortably and so that you have good access to the part to be treated.

  2. Expose the area to be treated, and do not apply modalities over clothes. Remember to be professional and respect the patient's modesty.

II. Applying the modality

A. Specifics of application will be presented in each section of this lab manual.

B. Familiarize yourself with each piece of equipment before treatment. Have access to instruction manuals and practice with specific machines before using them on patients.

C. Do not leave the athlete alone at any time during the treatment. The athlete should be able to discontinue treatment if necessary with an emergency shutoff switch.

III. Terminating treatment

A. Turn intensity controls to zero output, disconnect the patient, and turn off the power.

B. Return everything neatly. Do not wind electrical cables tightly, because this can bend and damage the wires, resulting in a short.

C. Inspect the skin, noting any mottling or skin eruptions. Mild redness is expected with some applications.

D. Evaluate subjective and objective findings after treatment.

IV. Documenting treatment

A. Note equipment used.

B. Note length and intensity of treatment.

C. Note subjective and objective findings as compared with those before the treatment.

Name_____   Date_____

Discussion Questions

1. Look up the Practice Act in your state and describe how it governs modality use for athletic trainers. Discuss and note below how your state compares with others.

2. List which modalities might cause a problem if used when there is cardiovascular compromise. What types of patients would raise concern? How could you recognize signs and symptoms of cardiovascular distress?

3. In small discussion groups, describe and note below how modality use would change when
   - you are traveling with a college athletic team,
   - you are in a high school athletic training room,
   - you are in a physical therapy outpatient clinic,
   - you are working in professional sports,
   - you are in an industrial setting, and
   - you are in a training camp, and the athletic trainer who normally cares for the Olympic or international athletes is not present.

Come together as a class to discuss your answers.

Activities

1. Explore the lab equipment that will be available for practice throughout this course. Identify the types of machines that are present. Note locations of modalities and other supplies that may be necessary such as towels, an ice machine, bags, and ultrasound gel.

2. Discuss the systematic method for modality application. Discuss professionalism and how it pertains to modality use in athletic training. Are there any modifications to this procedure in your setting? Complete a mock evaluation of an injury by running through the steps outlined in this lab. Note your findings in the space provided.

3. Show three safety concerns regarding modalities in your athletic training room and discuss how these might be rectified. Note your findings in the space provided.

LAB 2

Development of the Treatment Plan

Review material from chapter 1, pages 6 to 11 of the textbook, before you complete this lab.

OBJECTIVES

- You will understand the importance of an evaluation in developing a plan for modality use.

- You will be able to develop a problem list from the results of the evaluation.

- You will be able to determine short-term and long-term goals.

- You will be able to determine which modalities can address specific problems.

- You will be able to document modality use and the results of the treatment.

IMPORTANCE OF THE EVALUATION AND DEVELOPMENT OF THE PROBLEM LIST

The musculoskeletal evaluation should be thorough enough that the athletic trainer can generate a list of problems associated with the injury. When the athletic trainer bases the rehabilitation program on the problem list, the program is designed specifically for each athlete and modifications can be made throughout the plan. Although treatment guidelines and protocols are helpful to remind the athletic trainer of important issues with specific types of injuries, the problem-solving approach ensures that all key factors that are discovered in the evaluation are addressed with appropriate interventions.

The athletic trainer should use a systematic evaluation and begin listing problems. The subjective portion of the evaluation gives key information about limitations in function and pain; however, the athletic trainer should attempt to list the problems as objectively as possible. For example, pain should be described with respect to location, intensity, quality, frequency, and the provoking activity. Range of motion, strength, and swelling should be measured whenever possible. All aspects of the evaluation should be considered, including special tests, neuromuscular considerations such as atrophy or muscle tone, posture, end-feels, and proprioception. Function can be reported subjectively as a percentage: For example, the athlete is functioning at 65%. A more objective method of evaluating function is to measure something that the athlete does: for example, the athlete is able to run 30 min at a pace of 6 mph without pain or limping.

Once the problem list has been generated, the problems should be prioritized. For example, with a postoperative knee there may be loss of motion, loss of strength, and effusion. The effusion must be addressed first because this may prevent full motion. Additionally, strength cannot be addressed until neuromuscular control of the quadriceps has been restored. The athletic trainer should begin to think about which problems are linked so that the continuum of the rehabilitation program can be established. This leads to the formulation of short-term and long-term goals.

SHORT-TERM GOALS AND LONG-TERM GOALS

All treatments performed in the athletic training room should be justified by either short-term or long-term goals. This improves the accountability of the clinician, and the effectiveness of each treatment can be determined. The program should be reevaluated continually so that modifications can be made when necessary. Goal-oriented treatments prevent the excessive use of modalities because only treatments that can help meet the athlete's goals are used. Likewise, because each treatment is associated with a problem, the effectiveness of each treatment can be monitored more easily.

Short-term goals are difficult to determine and require practice and experience. Short-term goals are usually established for a 1- to 2-week period and are modified continually with progress and activity level. Commonly, an athlete or coach will ask when the athlete will be back to sports. For example, after a grade II ankle sprain, how long will the athlete be out? Many factors are used to formulate the timeline, but a goal-oriented approach keeps the focus on achievements. First, the athlete is told he or she can discard the crutches when able to walk comfortably without a limp. Running may begin when the athlete can walk briskly for 30 min without pain or swelling. Cutting, sprinting, and sport-specific activities begin when jogging is well tolerated. Each aspect of the program can be broken down in this manner. The short-term goals should be based on realistic expectations that depend on the severity of the injury and the level of dysfunction.

All goals should be realistic and objective so that it is clear when the athlete has met those goals. Each goal should have a measurable outcome with a specific time duration. The method used to achieve those goals becomes the rehabilitation plan.

Long-term goals are the final measurable outcome expected at the conclusion of rehabilitation. Again, these goals should be stated in a behavioral, objective manner so that it is clear that the goal has been achieved. Practicing in individual drills, sprinting a 4.4-sec 40-yard dash, or competing without restriction are long-term goals. Long-term goals are generally easy to write because they are the expected outcome of the rehabilitation. Putting a specific time frame on your expectation is more difficult, and expertise comes with practice.

Examples of Short-Term Goals for a Knee Injury

- Effusion should be reduced to no more than +2 cm girth in 1 week.
- The athlete should be able to perform eight sets of 10 straight-leg raises in 2 days with good quadriceps tone.
- The range of motion of the knee should be 0° to 130° in 1 week.
- The athlete should be able to perform body-weight 3/4 squats in 2 weeks.
- The athlete should be able to walk at 3.5 mph on the treadmill for 30 min in 10 days.

TREATMENTS

Treatments are directed by the short-term goals. The clinician should recognize what interventions can help meet the short-term goals, which may include activity modification, application of modalities, and therapeutic exercise. The appropriate use of each modality is discussed in following labs.

Knowing when to discontinue a treatment is just as important as knowing when to use a treatment. It is common for a new clinician to continue to add exercises or modalities as the patient progresses. Eventually the athlete spends 3 h in rehabilitation, which is not effective time management. The athletic trainer should reevaluate periodically, especially if a short-term goal has been met. The problem list can be modified, and it may become clear that a specific treatment is no longer necessary.

DOCUMENTATION

All treatments should be documented so that the treatment can be reproduced exactly by another clinician. Dosages of modalities such as ultrasound should be documented to include the frequency, intensity, duration, and duty cycle. Other factors, such as position of the athlete and locations of electrodes for electrical stimulation, should be documented as well.

Name_____   Date_____

Discussion Questions

1. The following list includes some common results of sports injuries. Determine and note below which can be addressed by the use of modalities. Discuss possibilities with each of the following problems. Note that some problems are addressed with other treatments, such as exercise! After discussing the following list, come together as a class and compile a list of all the possible treatments for each problem.

   - Decreased range of motion
   - Swelling (effusion or edema)
   - Pain
   - Neuromuscular inhibition
   - Loss of function
   - Loss of strength
   - Loss of proprioception
   - Inflammation (warmth and redness)
   - Ecchymosis
   - Muscle spasm

2. Note below methods to determine when to discontinue a particular treatment.

3. List the potential problems of using several modalities in the same treatment, for example, heat, ultrasound, massage, exercise, electrical stimulation, and ice. How will you be able to monitor the effects of one treatment compared with another?

4. If an athlete reports that he or she had more pain after the last treatment, note below what modifications can be made rather than changing the entire approach to managing the condition.

Activities

1. For each of the following patient case studies, create a problem list with goals. Note that all treatments should address the athlete's problems and that not all problems can be addressed with modalities (see table for an example of a problem list for Case A).

    Case A: A field hockey player sustained a plantar flexion, inversion ankle sprain. After reporting to the athletic training room, she has a moderate-sized hematoma on the lateral malleolus. There is intense pain (8 on a scale of 10) anterior and inferior to the lateral malleolus on palpation. There is no pain with palpation of the distal fibula, distal tibia, or base of the fifth metatarsal. The athlete has an antalgic gait. All motion causes pain.

Establishment of the Treatment Plan

Problems	Short-term goals	Treatment
Pain	Decrease pain to 5 on a scale of 10 in 24 h	Ice and transcutaneous electrical nerve stimulation
Hematoma	Decrease swelling to normal in 5 d	Ice/compression with horseshoe/elevation
Decreased range of motion	Increase range of motion (ROM) to normal in plantar flexion, eversion, and dorsiflexion in 5 d; increase ROM of inversion to normal in 1 wk	Ice/active ROM
Antalgic gait	Normal gait in 2 d	Crutches and gait training
	Long-term goals	
Loss of cardiovascular fitness	Pass fitness test before participation (1.5 miles in 12 min)	Cross training and interval training on stationary bike and in pool
Inability to perform (playing field hockey)	Play field hockey without pain or swelling in 2 wk	Progression from running, cutting, and individual drills to contact activities

The same player after 5 days of treatment continues to have decreased range of motion, especially into inversion. Gait is normal. Mild effusion remains, but the ankle is not warm to palpation. There is decreased strength in all planes and the ankle feels "weak".

Problems	Short-term goals	Treatment
	Long-term goals	

Case B: An 18-year-old baseball pitcher reports to the athletic training room with pain in the posterior aspect of the right shoulder, especially after throwing. On examination, you notice that he has rounded shoulders and general poor posture. He has excessive passive external rotation but reduced internal rotation of the right shoulder. He has pain with resisted motion of shoulder abduction and external rotation, but strength is good (5 on a scale of 5 in all shoulder motions). He describes the shoulder pain as dull and difficult to localize. There is a positive impingement sign and pain on palpation in the deep posterior aspect of the shoulder. He reports that he is functioning at about 90% due to pain.

Problems	Short-term goals	Treatment
	Long-term goals	

Case C: A basketball player reports that his knee has been swelling on occasion. The team is in the middle of the conference schedule and he is the starting point guard. On examination, there is no appreciable effusion, nor is there pain with hyperflexion. The joint line is not painful on palpation. There is marked pain with resisted knee extension, and the patellar tendon insertion is extremely painful on palpation. The athlete is able to function, although he reports pain and stiffness, especially at the beginning of practice.

Problems	Short-term goals	Treatment
	Long-term goals	

There are no "correct" answers for the previous case studies. There will be different interpretations and treatments even among classmates. The "practice" of athletic training implies that with more experience, a clinician can use information about similar cases to help formulate the appropriate treatments. However, you should have a systematic method of evaluation to ensure that you gather all relevant information.

Athletic trainers should be careful to not "do" everything for the athlete. The most important aspect of injury resolution is rehabilitation, and the athlete should understand that he or she must perform therapeutic exercise to rectify most problems. Modality application requires direct clinician intervention, whereas rehabilitative exercise should be done by the athlete with guided independence. As professionals, we do not want to create a dependency in which athletes need us to perform their entire treatment program for them. Athletic trainers should strive to direct the athlete's care and encourage the athlete to assume the ultimate responsibility for his or her health care.

LAB 3

Pain and
Pain Measurement

Review material from chapter 4, pages 46 to 71 of
the textbook, before you complete this lab.

OBJECTIVES

- You will understand normal pain transmission.

- You will explore methods of pain measurement.

- You will understand that minimizing pain is a primary goal of modality use so that therapeutic exercise can be initiated.

PAIN

Pain occurs to some degree with almost every athletic injury. Pain is beneficial because it allows the athlete to recognize that an injury has occurred and it prevents the athlete from continuing to stress the injury. Acute pain is well-localized and generally short-lived. If a basketball player sprains his ankle, he knows immediately. If the injury is minor, the pain generally subsides and he can return to play. If the injury is more severe, pain limits his function and the player is unable to continue. Once the extent of the injury is known, pain is a guide for therapeutic exercise. If the athlete has pain during an exercise, then the stress is too great. Exercise should always be at a level below the pain threshold.

Relieving pain is often a focus of therapeutic modalities. Pain during rest or beyond what is necessary to protect the athlete should be treated with medication, modalities, and activity modification. The goal is to reduce pain so that therapeutic exercise can be performed. Heat, ice, ultrasound, electrical stimulation, and mechanical therapies all have the capacity to reduce pain. Therapeutic modalities including transcutaneous electrical nerve stimulation (TENS) and ice are intended to reduce pain but do not eliminate pain or sensory function.

Acute pain is the most common in athletic injuries and usually resolves over time regardless of the treatment. Chronic pain or persistent pain, however, is much more difficult to treat. Persistent pain continues past any usefulness. Many clinicians use the arbitrary time delineation of greater than 6 weeks when describing chronic pain, because most acute injuries resolve in this time frame. Pain is a multifaceted experience that affects numerous brain centers. Persistent pain may be the result of the propitiation of certain neural pathways. Ultimately the affective–motivational component of the pain experience affects the physical, emotional, and social well-being of the patient or athlete.

Referred pain occurs when there is pain in another area separate from the pathology. Examples of referred pain are when the left arm and jaw become painful during a heart attack or when there is left shoulder pain with a spleen injury. Unlike the skin and soft tissue, the viscera have very few sensory organs. When the sensory information synapses at the spinal cord, interneurons are activated at that level. The interneurons converge on the neurons that localize pain to the dermatome or myotome at the same spinal cord level. The brain interprets the pain as arising from the soft tissues rather than the involved organ. A thorough evaluation of the injury should identify the area of pathology so that the injury is treated rather than the pain site.

Radiating pain is another type of pain that is difficult to evaluate and treat. Radiating pain generally comes from an injured nerve or nerve root and is perceived in a different area than the location of the pathology. For example, when there is a lumbar disc injury with pressure on a nerve root, pain, paresthesia, or numbness is felt in the back of the thigh or in the leg. Proper evaluation is essential to determine the site of pathology.

ANATOMY IN PAIN TRANSMISSION

To understand normal pain transmission and pain modulation, a basic overview of nerve fibers is necessary. Nerve fibers also are classified by their function: pain, sensory, or motor. The largest nerve fibers are the A fibers, which are the fastest conducting motor and sensory nerve fibers. This group is subdivided into A-alpha, A-beta, A-gamma, and A-delta, depending on their size. These larger nerve fibers have a low capacitance and are the most quickly stimulated.

The B fibers are smaller myelinated fibers and are generally the efferent fibers of the autonomic nervous system. These fibers usually are not associated with direct responses of electrical stimulation but may act indirectly as an important link between some of the physiological effects of electrical stimulation.

The C fibers are unmyelinated and include the efferent postganglionic fibers of the sympathetic nervous system and the smallest afferent peripheral nerves, which usually are associated with pain. The C fibers are the slowest in conduction and take more stimulation to elicit a response. Because the A and C fibers have sensory components, they play the largest role in both pain and pain control. Many pain control theories and electrical-stimulation protocols use the properties of these nerve fibers to produce their response.

NORMAL PAIN TRANSMISSION

Understanding normal pain transmission is imperative to understanding pain modulation theories. The key anatomy and physiology of normal pain transmission are described next. Pain is transmitted systematically from the injured area to the brain. Acute pain is a rapid, three-neuron sequence to provide accurate information about the location of injury. The nociceptor is the sensory organ in the tissues that is sensitized to the painful stimulation. The information travels to the spinal cord via the sensory nerve. This fiber is known as the first-order neuron and may be either an A-delta or C fiber depending on the stimulus. All sensory nerve fibers have their cell bodies in the dorsal root ganglia and synapse in the spinal cord in the dorsal horn. The second-order neuron crosses to the opposite side of the spinal cord (decussates) and transmits the information up to the thalamus. The second-order neuron commonly is termed the *T-cell*, although pain usually is carried by the lateral spinothalamic tract. At the thalamus, there is a synapse onto the third-order neuron, which carries information to the sensory cortex of the brain, where the pain is acknowledged. The three-neuron pathway describes the neospinothalamic system:

1. Nociceptor (in the skin, soft tissue, and periosteum).
2. Sensory nerve (cell body is in the dorsal root ganglion and synapses in the dorsal horn of the spinal cord).
3. T-cell: Second-order neuron that "transmits" a signal to the thalamus. The name *T-cell* is given to this neuron because pain, temperature, light touch, vibration, and deep touch are carried on different tracts. Therefore, *T-cell* is a generic name for the second-order neuron.
4. Thalamus: Second-order neuron synapses here with the third-order neuron. This area also sends information to emotion centers of the brain, which causes some of the typical responses to a pain sensation.
5. Sensory cortex: Area of the brain that identifies the location of pain (see figure 3.1).

PAIN MODULATION

Almost every patient will have pain on his or her problem list, so the effective measurement and treatment of pain are essential in caring for the injury. Pain, however, is a complex entity that involves neuroanatomy and neurophysiology as well as pharmacology. Sports medicine clinicians have several methods of treating pain with therapeutic modalities. Figures 3.2 through 3.4 (pp. 19-20) represent some of the current theories on pain modulation. Understanding the fundamentals of the pain modulation theories is essential in learning to use the different types of electrical stimulation and other pain management modalities. The pain modulation theories are categorized by the level of the central nervous system that is targeted. For example, the sensory level pain modulation theory targets the structures in the spinal cord, the noxious level

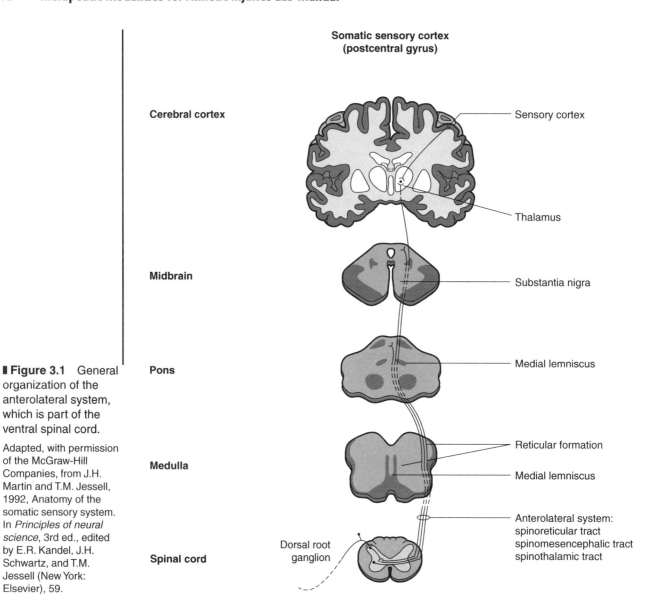

Somatic sensory cortex
(postcentral gyrus)

Cerebral cortex — Sensory cortex

Thalamus

Midbrain — Substantia nigra

Pons — Medial lemniscus

Medulla — Reticular formation

Medial lemniscus

Anterolateral system:
spinoreticular tract
spinomesencephalic tract
spinothalamic tract

Dorsal root
ganglion

Spinal cord

■ Figure 3.1 General organization of the anterolateral system, which is part of the ventral spinal cord.

Adapted, with permission of the McGraw-Hill Companies, from J.H. Martin and T.M. Jessell, 1992, Anatomy of the somatic sensory system. In *Principles of neural science*, 3rd ed., edited by E.R. Kandel, J.H. Schwartz, and T.M. Jessell (New York: Elsevier), 59.

targets the brainstem, and the motor level targets higher brain centers. These pain modulation theories have numerous names, but the current terminology (*sensory, noxious,* and *motor*) is used to describe the type of stimulation that modulates pain.

Gate Theory (Sensory Level Pain Modulation) (Melzack and Wall 1965)

The sensory level pain modulation theory targets the structures in the spinal cord. The A-beta fibers are the large-diameter sensory fibers of the skin. When they are stimulated, the substantia gelatinosa is activated (figure 3.2). The substantia gelatinosa acts as a presynaptic inhibitor that modulates pain by terminating presynaptically upon the large and small fibers just before their termination on the T-cells. When the substantia gelatinosa is active, the presynaptic inhibition increases (gate is closed). Input from the small-diameter A-delta and C fibers is prevented from traveling to the brain. Ultimately, less sensory stimulation is perceived by the T-cell. The idea that A-beta fibers could "close the gate" resulted in the development of TENS units to modulate pain perception.

These neuroanatomic structures include

- A-beta fibers,

- A-delta and C fibers,
- substantia gelatinosa, and
- transmission cells (T-cells).

It was proposed later, in 1972, that an interneuron that used enkephalin (a naturally occurring opiate) was present in the area known as the substantia gelatinosa (figure 3.3). This led to the revised model of the gate theory.

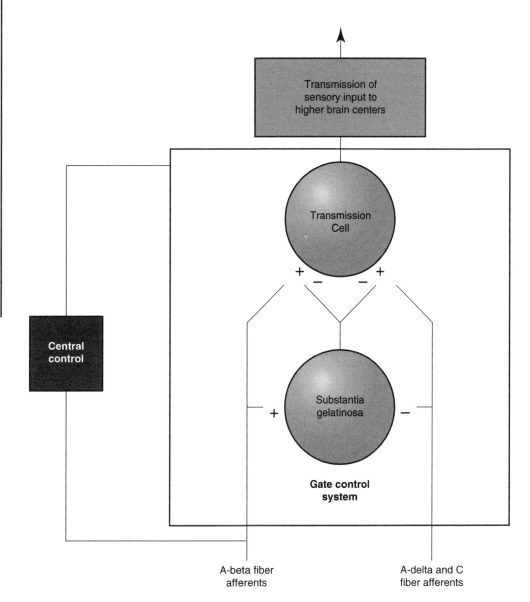

▌Figure 3.2 The gate control theory. Input along large-diameter (A-beta) primary afferents activates inhibitory influence of substantia gelatinosa on transmission from primary to afferent nerves to a transmission cell (second-order afferent).

Reprinted, by permission, from C.R. Denegar, 2000, *Therapeutic modalities for athletic injuries* (Champaign, IL: Human Kinetics), 63.

Noxious Pain Modulation

Noxious pain theory operates on the idea that pain inhibits pain. When a controlled, noxious stimulation is applied, areas in the brain become active and emit neurochemicals to reduce the pain. Noxious pain modulation utilizes descending control of pain (figure 3.4), since the impact of pain has already reached the higher brain centers and the neurochemicals act at lower levels of the central nervous system (i.e., segmental spinal level).

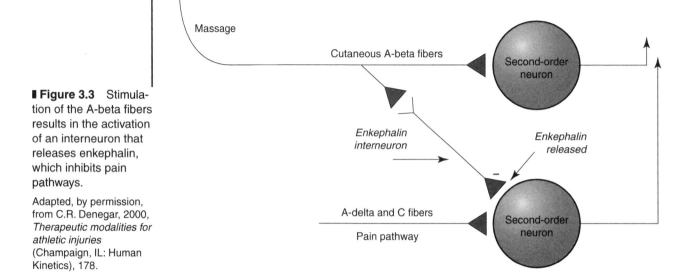

Massage

Cutaneous A-beta fibers

Second-order neuron

Enkephalin interneuron →

Enkephalin released

–

A-delta and C fibers

Pain pathway

Second-order neuron

■ Figure 3.3 Stimulation of the A-beta fibers results in the activation of an interneuron that releases enkephalin, which inhibits pain pathways.

Adapted, by permission, from C.R. Denegar, 2000, *Therapeutic modalities for athletic injuries* (Champaign, IL: Human Kinetics), 178.

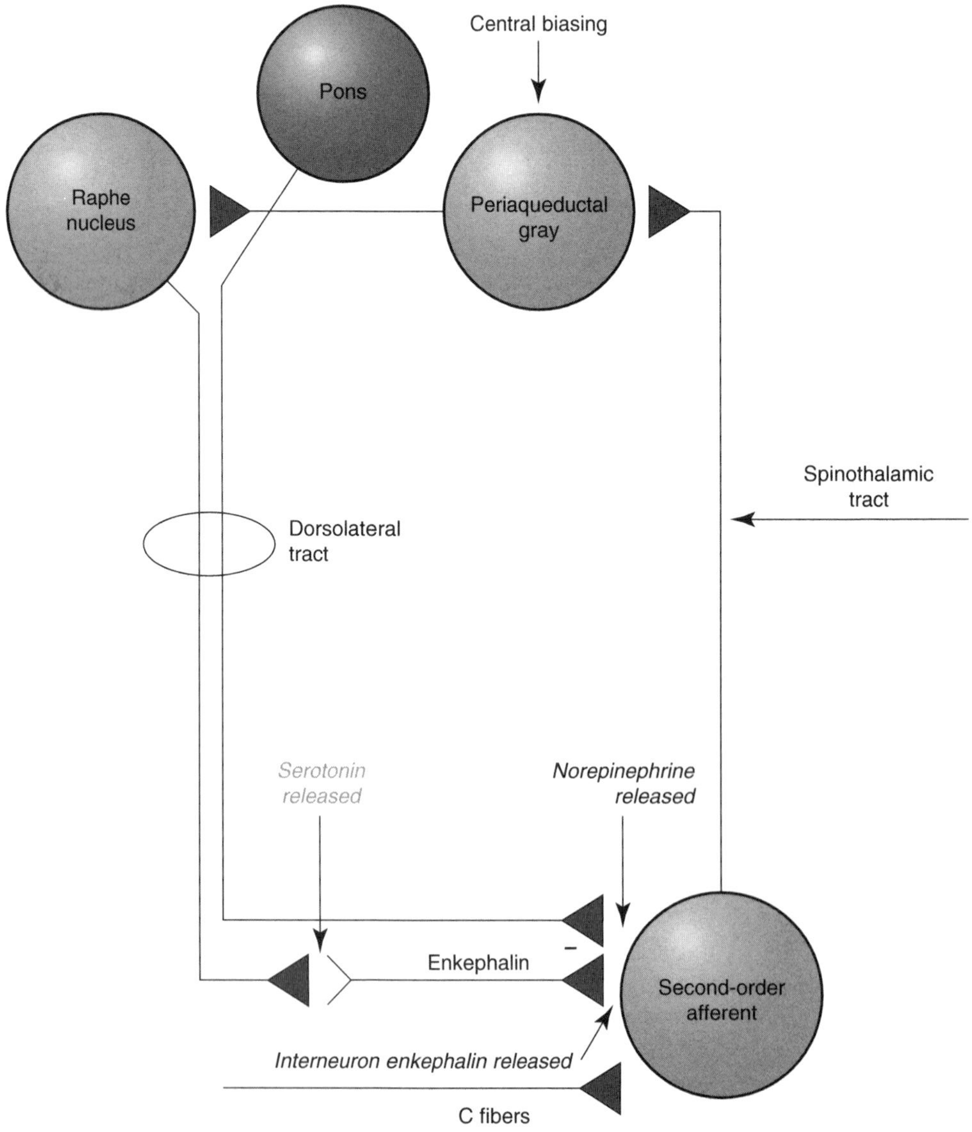

Central biasing

Pons

Raphe nucleus

Periaqueductal gray

Spinothalamic tract

Dorsolateral tract

Serotonin released

Norepinephrine released

Enkephalin

–

Second-order afferent

Interneuron enkephalin released

C fibers

■ Figure 3.4 Noxious theory of pain control.

Adapted, by permission, from C.R. Denegar, 2000, *Therapeutic modalities for athletic injuries* (Champaign, IL: Human Kinetics), 66.

Neuroanatomic structures used in noxious level pain modulation include

- C-fiber,
- central nervous system connections,
- periaquaductal gray area (PAG), and
- raphe nucleus (nucleus raphe magnus).

This type of pain modulation has been examined since the 1960s, when a researcher noted that stimulation of the PAG produced analgesia in unanesthetized rats. The raphe nucleus tends to preferentially inhibit A-delta (over A-beta) fibers and contains serotonin-carrying neurons. Serotonergic neurons are concentrated heavily in lamina I of the dorsal horn of the spinal cord and are presumed to have a direct monosynaptic inhibitory effect on the second-order neuron (ascending tract neuron, or T-cell).

A second system that originates in the pons also produces dorsal horn inhibition and analgesia. The descending inhibitory system may terminate directly on second-order neurons (T-cells) or indirectly via an enkephalinergic interneuron.

This conceptual model is "turned on" by eliciting pain (C fibers) in the affected region. The clinician can use certain types of electrical stimulation to excite C fibers.

Motor Level Pain Control

Motor level pain control targets the higher brain centers and is pain control through endorphins and adrenocorticotropic hormones (ACTH). Endorphins are part of a complex neurophysiological system that decreases pain. They are naturally produced (endogenous) opiates that are produced in the central nervous system. The goal of motor pain modulation is to enhance the production of endorphins. No TENS treatment can eliminate pain, but if the pain is decreased, even temporarily, therapeutic exercise can be initiated. Exercise, along with other pain-relieving therapies such as joint mobilization and passive range of motion, can help resolve the cycle of pain and spasm. Neuroanatomic structures include

- A-delta fibers,
- beta lipotropins and endorphins, and
- ACTH.

Endorphins are produced primarily in the anterior pituitary through the breakdown of a large molecular complex known as beta-lipotropin. The beta-lipotropin molecule is broken down to produce beta-endorphin and certain types of enkephalins that have strong analgesic qualities. ACTH also is produced in the pituitary gland and may affect cortisol production from the adrenal glands that lie superior to the kidneys. Variations in cortisol production are normal, and subtle changes in ACTH levels are difficult to measure (figure 3.5).

The endogenous opiate production is theorized to be enhanced by the low-frequency, high-intensity stimulation of peripheral nerve fibers. The frequency of stimulation must be in the range of 2 to 7 cycles per second at intensities sufficient to evoke muscular contraction. Furthermore, endorphin also has been shown to exert a powerful influence on the raphe nucleus and PAG, which activate the descending control system. Therefore, when motor pain modulation is elicited with rhythmic muscle contractions, along with A-delta fibers, noxious pain modulation (descending tract) is enhanced as well.

Low-frequency stimulation of trigger and acupuncture points is very valuable in treating chronic and acute pain and injury. Increased corticosteroid levels from the enhanced ACTH production provide analgesic effects as well. Enhancement of

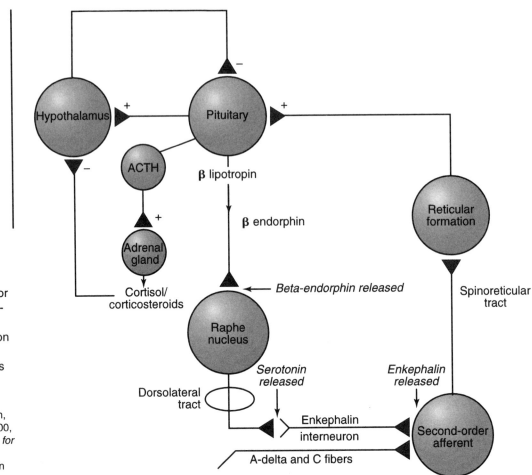

■ Figure 3.5 Motor level pain control. Neuroanatomic structures are stimulated by pulsed, motor stimulation to elicit A-delta fiber excitation. Motor pain modulation requires strong but tolerable contractions at 2 to 7 pulses per second (pps).

Adapted, by permission, from C.R. Denegar, 2000, *Therapeutic modalities for athletic injuries* (Champaign, IL: Human Kinetics), 67.

pituitary production of hormonal and analgesic factors also may account for the success of low-frequency TENS.

PAIN MEASUREMENT METHODS

It is important to develop techniques to quantify the pain experience. This helps to determine whether a patient is making progress and it gives information about the effectiveness of the treatment. Pain measurement should be reliable and valid, which is difficult because of the subjective nature of pain. The following sections describe common pain measurement techniques in athletic training.

VISUAL ANALOGUE SCALE

The visual analogue scale is a 10-cm line with no demarcations (so that the athlete will not remember where he or she marked the last scale) (see figure 3.6). On the left end are the words *no pain* and on the right end *intolerable pain*, which should imply postsurgical or excruciating pain. The clinician measures in millimeters the horizontal distance from the left to the athlete's mark of the extent of his or her pain. This type of measure attempts to make pain more of an objective measure, even though it remains subjective.

No pain   Intolerable pain

∎ Figure 3.6 The visual analogue scale.

VERBAL PAIN RATING

The verbal pain rating is used to quickly assess the intensity of the athlete's pain. The athlete reports on a scale from 0 to 10 how painful the condition is; 0 represents no pain and 10 represents intolerable pain. This test becomes less effective when the athlete is asked for a score several times throughout the evaluation and treatment. For example, the athlete will remember reporting a 5 before the treatment and will use that as a reference for reporting his or her score after the treatment is over.

PQRST RATING

To determine the qualitative experience of pain, use the PQRST acronym. All questions should be open-ended, and "yes or no" questions should be avoided. *P* stands for provocation—how did the injury occur and what makes it better or worse? *Q* stands for quality—what does the pain feel like? *R* stands for referral or radiation—does the pain appear to follow a dermatome or pattern? *S* stands for severity—quantify the pain. *T* stands for timing—when does it hurt?

MCGILL PAIN QUESTIONNAIRE

This measure attempts to both quantify and qualify pain. The athlete uses a body diagram to demonstrate the extent of the pain, which is helpful in understanding radiating pain or pain syndromes. Additionally, the athlete identifies certain adjectives to describe the type of pain, which can help the clinician understand the cause of the pain (e.g., an aggravated nerve root vs. a compression injury to the soft tissue or bruise). Finally, the McGill Pain Questionnaire ends with a visual analogue scale to help quantify the intensity of the pain (see form 3.1).

Form 3.1 McGill Pain Questionnaire

Part 1: Using the diagram, draw the location of the pain. Indicate whether the pain is internal or external using an I or E. Indicate with an IE when the pain is both internal and external.

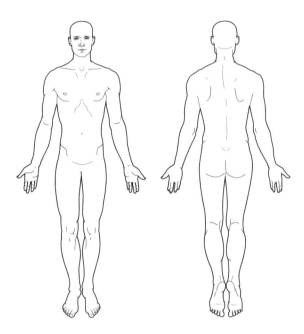

Reprinted, by permission, from P. Houglum, 2001, *Therapeutic exercise for athletic injuries* (Champaign, IL: Human Kinetics), 169.

Part 2: What does your pain feel like?

Some of the words below describe your present pain. Circle only those words that best describe it. Leave out any category that is not suitable. Use only a single word in each appropriate category—the one that applies best.

1	2	3	4	5
Flickering	Jumping	Pricking	Sharp	Pinching
Quivering	Flashing	Boring	Cutting	Pressing
Pulsing	Shooting	Drilling	Lacerating	Gnawing
Throbbing		Stabbing		Cramping
Beating		Lancinating		Crushing
Pounding				

6	7	8	9	10
Tugging	Hot	Tingling	Dull	Tender
Pulling	Burning	Itchy	Sore	Taut
Wrenching	Scalding	Smarting	Hurting	Rasping
	Searing	Stinging	Aching	Splitting
			Heavy	

11	12	13	14	15
Tiring	Sickening	Fearful	Punishing	Wretched
Exhausting	Suffocating	Frightful	Grueling	Blinding
		Terrifying	Cruel	
			Vicious	
			Killing	
16	**17**	**18**	**19**	**20**
Annoying	Spreading	Tight	Cool	Nagging
Troublesome	Radiating	Numb	Cold	Nauseating
Miserable	Penetrating	Drawing	Freezing	Agonizing
Intense	Piercing	Squeezing		Dreadful
Unbearable		Tearing		Torturing

The adjectives used to describe pain enlighten the clinician about the athlete's pain—the cause, frequency, and type as well as how the athlete is dealing with the pain. The McGill Pain Questionnaire is used to treat the multifaceted qualities of pain and can help identify strategies to deal with the problem.

Part 3: How does your pain change with time?

   A. Which word or words would you use to describe the pattern of your pain?

   B. What kind of things relieve your pain?

   C. What kind of things increase your pain?

Part 4: How strong is your pain?

People agree that the following words represent pain of increasing intensity.

1	2	3	4	5
Mild	Discomforting	Distressing	Horrible	Excruciating

To answer the following questions, write the number of the most appropriate word in the space beside the question.

   1. Which word describes your pain right now?

   2. Which word describes it at its worst?

   3. Which word describes it when it is least?

   4. Which word describes the worst toothache you ever had?

   5. Which word describes the worst headache you ever had?

   6. Which word describes the worst stomachache you ever had?

© 1984, 1970 by R. Melzack. Adapted by permission.

Name_____   Date_____

Discussion Questions

1. How would you summarize your findings from the McGill Pain Questionnaire? This method of evaluating pain considers many intangible aspects of pain and commonly is reserved for use with chronic-pain patients. Would this assessment tool be beneficial in athletic training?

2. Discuss the following with respect to the injuries that you have treated. Note below how you could recognize each type.
   - Acute pain

   - Chronic pain

   - Somatic pain

   - Referred pain

   - Radiating pain

   - Night pain

Activities

1. In small groups, draw schematics of pain transmission
   - Gate theory—sensory pain modulation

   - Noxious pain modulation (descending tract)

   - Motor pain modulation

2. Practice using the PQRST technique of pain evaluation for the following examples:
   - Anterior cruciate ligament tear
   - Sprained ankle
   - Herniated disc at L 5/S 1
   - Plantar fasciitis
   - Impingement syndrome in the shoulder
   - Cervical and thoracic spasm with headaches

3. To create a model to assess pain in a lab situation, demonstrate the cold pressor test to evoke pain. Fill a container with ice and water so that the temperature is 40° F. Have a volunteer place his or her nondominant hand into the water. At each minute, record the intensity of pain by using a visual analogue scale. Repeat with another subject and record pain by using the verbal rating scale. Discuss the pain measures with respect to their objectivity and accuracy; note your findings in the space provided.

LAB 4

Therapeutic Cold Application

Review material from chapter 7, pages 100 to 121 of the textbook, before you complete this lab.

OBJECTIVES

- You will understand the types of cold therapies available and how they are applied.

- You will be able to determine the duration for cold application depending on the location of the injury.

- You will be able to determine when cold application is indicated.

- You will understand the contraindications and precautions for cold therapy.

- You will understand cryokinetics and when and how this treatment is applied.

Cold therapy, or cryotherapy, is the modality most commonly used by athletic trainers. Athletic trainers are generally present at the event in which the injury occurs, so they see the injury and can evaluate it before spasm and swelling ensue. Following the evaluation on the sideline, the immediate application of ice, compression, and elevation helps to control bleeding and prevent secondary cell death by hypoxia. Cryotherapy controls the inflammatory process that occurs with all injuries. Inflammation cannot be stopped, and the process is necessary to allow for healing and repair to occur; however, the by-products of inflammation, such as swelling and pain, can cause further debilitation.

Ice delays or minimizes swelling, decreases pain, and decreases muscle spasm, thus limiting the magnitude of injury. Lowering tissue temperature causes a local vasoconstriction, reduces capillary permeability due to the lessened effect of chemical mediators, and makes the blood more viscous. All of those processes decrease blood flow to the injured area, which can reduce swelling.

The exact mechanism with which ice dulls peripheral pain is not known. However, lowering tissue temperature interferes locally with nerve impulses and decreases nerve conduction velocity. Ice relieves spasm by decreasing muscle activity and muscle spindle firing. Ice limits the magnitude of tissue damage by lowering the metabolism of adjacent uninjured cells. The cooler temperature decreases the cellular demand for oxygen for healthy cells, which increases their survival rate while local circulation is disrupted.

Ice may be applied as soon as possible after the injury for 20 to 30 min to allow good penetration. The deeper the injured structure, the longer the ice application. For example, a deep thigh bruise may require 40 min of ice therapy to effectively cool the tissue, whereas a finger may require only 5 to 10 min. It is not possible to prevent all hematomas because of frank bleeding in severe injuries. However, ice helps minimize swelling. Ice also can be applied over a compression bandage postoperatively to manage pain and swelling, but longer durations of application are necessary.

CRYOTHERAPY APPLICATION

An athletic trainer has several options for therapeutic cold application. The most common are described here, along with instructions for their application and the optimal duration of treatment. With all cryotherapy application, explain to the athlete that he or she will perceive four sensations: cold, burning, aching, and then numbness or analgesia. Analgesia should occur in 5 to 7 min of constant application.

ICE PACKS

Ice packs are inexpensive and readily available for most athletic events. Ice packs are made from ice placed in a plastic bag. They are most effective when crushed ice is used, because this conforms to the tissues. All air should be eliminated from the bag because air acts as an insulator. Too much ice in the bag prevents the ice from conforming to nonuniform body parts (see figure 4.1).

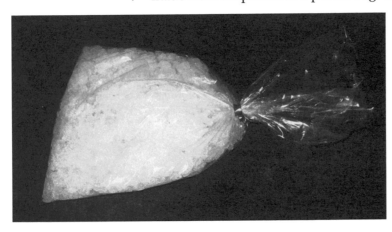

■ **Figure 4.1**   A plastic bag should be partially filled with crushed ice. Air should be eliminated from the bag, and it should be either tied or sealed near the top.

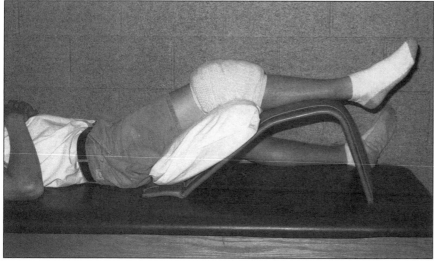

To apply the ice pack, make the ice bag and position the athlete appropriately. Expose the area to be treated; the ice pack should not be applied over clothing. Because a dry interface prevents adequate cooling of the body part, moisten a towel with warm water on one end and wrap it around the bag so that the moistened side is on the skin. When swelling is a concern, elevate the extremity above the level of the heart for the duration of the treatment (see figure 4.2).

■ Figure 4.2
Ice-compression-elevation: Position limb above heart and use elastic wrap with crushed ice.

COMMERCIAL COLD PACKS

Commercial cold packs often are used in clinics or athletic training rooms where there is access to a freezer. The benefits of these cold packs are that the gel easily conforms to the body and there is no danger of dripping cold water on the athlete. Cold packs such as Col Pac are chemical gel mixtures encased in vinyl. They are stored in a freezer unit between –5 and 5° C (around 32° F). They may take 1 to 2 h to recool after using. Other commercial cold packs use bladders filled with frozen water. Many shapes and sizes are available to conveniently use on different joints.

To use a commercial cold pack, remove it from the freezer and cover with one layer of warm, moist towel. This interface is for sanitary reasons and to increase the effectiveness of conduction. The interface can prevent injury as well, because these packs may be stored in a freezer that is colder than 0° C, which can cause frostbite to the skin. Apply the cold pack to the surface area, contouring the area to be treated. The treatment time is 15 to 45 min depending on the depth of the target tissue (see figure 4.3).

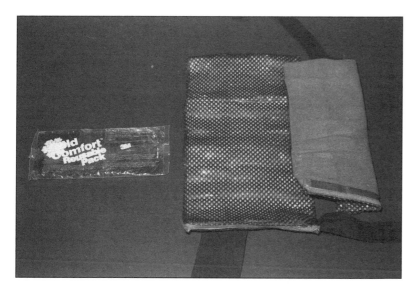

■ Figure 4.3 Commercial cold packs vary from gel to plastic cells that hold water. An interface should be used for hygiene and to prevent frostbite to the skin.

ICE MASSAGE

An ice massage is performed by using water frozen in a Styrofoam or paper cup, making this an inexpensive treatment for home use. Circular or linear motions are used to cover an area no greater than two or three times the surface of the ice. For larger treatment areas, a different type of cryotherapy must be used. Benefits of ice massage are the ease of home use, the pressure of massaging (which can help with pain relief), and the shorter length of time necessary for an effective treatment than with other methods of cryotherapy. Disadvantages are the mess from the melting ice and the limitation that ice massage is only effective for small treatment areas.

To apply an ice massage, position the athlete appropriately with a towel or draping to prevent water from dripping on either the patient or the treatment area. The top of the cup should be torn away to expose the ice. Using your hand, melt the outer layer of the ice cup to remove sharp edges. Apply the ice cup, keeping it constantly moving in the designated area. Expect that the skin will blanch or lose color with pressure. If raised areas occur during or after the treatment, the patient is hypersensitive to cold and the treatment should be discontinued. Redness occurs normally as the ice is removed (see figure 4.4).

Analgesia should occur in 10 min or less, which completes the treatment. The shorter treatment time is a result of the small area to be treated and the pressure associated with the massage, which temporarily decreases the cutaneous blood flow to the area.

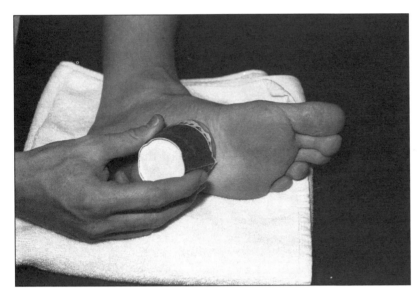

■ Figure 4.4 Ice massage should be limited to an area no more than two times the size of the cup.

COLD SUBMERSION

Cold submersion is a treatment used for a local application to the hand or foot. Although the limb must be in a dependent position during the treatment, this mode delivers circumferential and complete cooling to the extremity. Active exercise can be done with this mode, which promotes range of motion and contributes to edema resorption.

Fill a bucket or whirlpool with cold water and ice at a temperature ranging from 55 to 65° F. If a thermometer is not available, ice should be melting in the water. Ice slurry mixtures should be avoided because they are extremely noxious and do not provide any added benefit. Cold whirlpools move the water, which helps to control the temperature; however, the agitation should not cause discomfort. Immerse the area to be treated. Because it is impossible to combine an ice bath with elevation, the extremity can be wrapped with a single layer of wet elastic wrap to provide some compression during the treatment. A neoprene toe-cap can be used to protect the digits from the cold. Active range of motion in a pain-free range is encouraged. Treatment time should last 15 to 20 min (see figure 4.5).

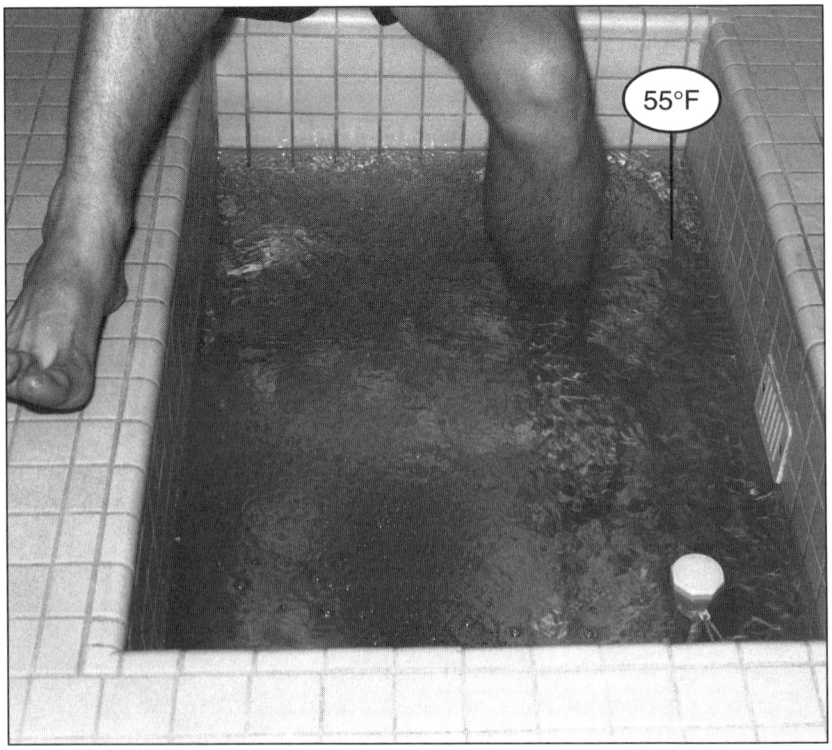

55°F

■ Figure 4.5 Cold water at a temperature of 55° F to 65° F should be used for cold submersion. This technique requires the extremity to be in a dependent position. However, active ROM is encouraged during the treatment.

CRYOKINETICS

Cryokinetics is the combination of cold therapy and exercise. The cold treatment decreases pain and helps to control the mild inflammatory response caused by therapeutic exercise. Although pain relief and numbness are associated with cryotherapy, sensation is not eliminated, so that the protective function of pain still exists. In other words, if the athlete cannot bend the knee without pain, ice treatment will not cause anesthesia to the joint to permit full range of motion. However, more motion will be permitted, which helps the return of neuromuscular function and early stress adaptation of collagen.

Cryokinetics involves the application of cold therapy, usually with an ice bag with range of motion exercise or ice submersion with active range of motion. The athlete should stay within the pain-free range for all exercise.

The classic technique of cryokinetics was described by Knight (1995). The injured part is thoroughly cooled with a 15- to 20-min cryotherapy treatment. The athlete follows the ice treatment by performing pain-free exercise such as gait training or mild resistance until mild discomfort returns (usually about 5 min).

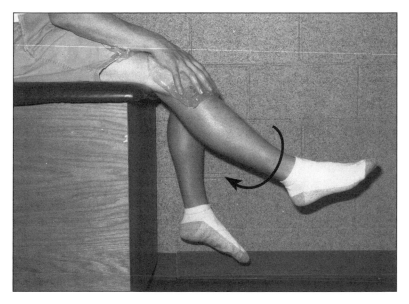

❚ Figure 4.6
Cryokinetics involves the combination of ice and exercise. In this example, the athlete uses ice to promote active range of motion to the knee.

The ice treatment is repeated for 5 min, and then the exercise routine is repeated. The exercise and ice treatment are alternated every 5 min for a total of 20 min. For example, with an ankle injury the limb is submerged for 10 to 15 min until analgesia sets in. The athlete then performs active exercise, including gait training if indicated, for about 5 min or until mild discomfort returns. The ankle is resubmerged for another 5 min to induce analgesia. This sequence is repeated for four cycles, and then the ankle is iced with elevation to prevent swelling (figure 4.6).

CRYOTHERAPY INDICATIONS

An athletic trainer needs to know when cryotherapy is indicated as a therapeutic modality. When an athlete experiences the following, cryotherapy is called for:

- Inflammation
- Pain
- Postoperative conditions
- Postexercise inflammation

However, there are times an athletic trainer must avoid cryotherapy. If the following are evident, do not use this modality:

- Decreased circulation (diabetic or cardiac conditions)
- Raynaud's phenomenon, a condition that causes vasospasm in the extremities and is exacerbated by cold
- Cold hypersensitivity or cold allergy

Additionally, use caution over superficial nerves such as the peroneal nerve at the knee and the ulnar nerve at the elbow.

Name_____ Date_____

Activities

1. In groups, practice setting up a volunteer with an ice pack, commercial cold pack, ice massage, and cold submersion. Note the time at which each sensation of cold, burning, aching, and numbness occurs with each treatment.

2. At the same time, place an ice pack on the dorsal aspect of your wrist and on your anterior thigh. Test for numbness after 5, 10, 15, and 20 min, and note results. Is your thigh completely cooled after 20 min?

3. For the following examples, describe and demonstrate the cold therapy application. Discuss and note the length of treatment.
   - Ankle sprain that occurred less than 1 h ago
   - Same ankle sprain 2 days later that has mild swelling but poor range of motion
   - Patellar tendinitis
   - Low back pain
   - Finger sprain
   - Knee sprain following rehabilitative exercise
   - Medial elbow pain in a pitcher

4. In small groups, choose a subject. Measure the length of time your subject can balance on one leg with his or her eyes closed. Submerge the subject's ankle for 20 min in 60° F water. Immediately measure the length of time he or she can balance on that leg with the eyes closed. Does ice treatment immediately affect proprioception or balance? Retest each 15 min to see if balance is affected as the ankle rewarms. Would this affect how you would manage an injury during practice or a game? Note your results.

LAB 5

Superficial Heat Application

Review material from chapter 7, pages 113 to 123 of the textbook, before you complete this lab.

OBJECTIVES

- You will understand the types of superficial heat therapies available and how they are applied.

- You will be able to determine the duration of superficial heat application depending on the location of the injury and the depth of the target tissue.

- You will understand when contrast therapy is indicated, how it is applied, and what physiological effects can be expected.

- You will be able to determine when superficial heat application is indicated.

- You will understand the contraindications and precautions for superficial heat therapy.

Heat is used during rehabilitation both to prepare the athlete for exercise and to increase flexibility when combined with a stretch. Superficial heat provides a mild inflammatory action and should not be used with acute injuries. Both ice and heat are analgesic agents, and both can reduce muscle spasm when used at the appropriate time during rehabilitation. Heat often is preferred by the athlete because of its sedating effects, but ice is more effective when the athlete complains of pain, not tightness, in the injured area.

Physiologically, superficial heat causes vasodilation from a sensory reflex, which increases blood flow to the skin. Superficial heat is most effective when combined with exercise. Heat increases the extensibility of connective tissue, but changes in range of motion can be achieved only when the tissue is stretched while the temperature is increased. It is also proposed that increases in intramuscular temperatures can decrease the chance of muscle injury. Superficial heat, however, has a depth of penetration of only 1 cm, which is unlikely to increase muscle temperature. The limitation in the depth of penetration is due to vasodilation, which increases blood flow and dissipates heat.

APPLICATION OF SUPERFICIAL HEAT

There are many methods of applying superficial heat, including hot packs, paraffin, fluidotherapy, and hydrotherapy. All types of superficial heat are limited to a penetration depth of about 1 cm, depending on the thickness of the layer of subcutaneous tissue. Treatment times vary with the structure to be treated, but it generally takes about 20 min for the tissues to reach therapeutic temperatures. Superficial areas such as the hands do not require as long a treatment.

HOT PACKS OR HYDROCOLLATOR PACKS

Hot packs or hydrocollator packs provide a superficial, moist heat. These commercial packs consist of a silica gel encased in canvas and are available in a variety of sizes. When not in use, the packs are stored in a stainless steel unit that contains hot water (150-170° F), which deters bacteria growth. The water temperature should be monitored regularly. Refer to the instruction manual if the temperature is not in the desired range. The thermostat should be calibrated yearly. The packs should be completely covered with water when stored, and fresh water may need to be added daily because of evaporation. Packs should be discarded when the silica gel begins to leak through the canvas covering. Clouding of water may indicate damaged or worn packs. The unit should be drained and cleaned at regular intervals. The stainless steel can be scrubbed with a nonabrasive detergent.

The actual temperature of the hot pack treatment ultimately is controlled by the number of towel layers used, rather than the temperature of the unit. Take care to avoid burning yourself by removing packs from the unit with metal tongs. Wrap packs with six to eight layers of toweling between the pack and the surface of the body. Commercial pack covers can be used but often require extra layers of toweling. Towels decrease the possibility of burning and keep the pack covers clean.

After determining that hot pack treatment is indicated, prepare the patient. Expose the area to be treated so that hot packs are not applied over clothing. The position of the athlete is very important for hot pack application. Heat increases extensibility of tissues, but only if the tissue is stretched during or immediately after the treatment. If possible, the athlete should be in a stretched position during the treatment. Adequate blood flow is required for heat dissipation, and areas of increased pressure may become ischemic; therefore, the athlete should not sit or lie on hot packs. Apply the pack to the treatment area, making sure the size of the pack is adequate. An extra large pack or two packs may be necessary to treat a large surface.

Explain that the athlete should perceive a sensation of warmth but not burning. Many people erroneously think "the hotter the better," which can result in burns.

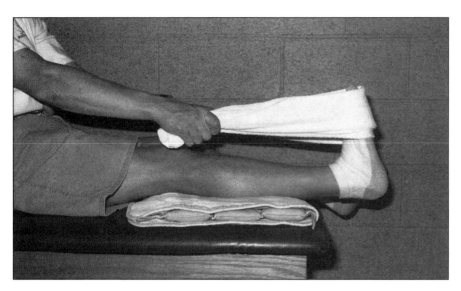

Check the athlete after about 5 min of application, applying or removing towels as appropriate. Check also for mottling erythema or patchy redness. If this is severe, discontinue treatment. Treatment time usually lasts 20 to 30 min. After removal, inspect the athlete's skin for burns. Mottled erythema might be present, which looks like patches of red and white. Continue to monitor the skin if this occurs since a more uniform redness is expected. Document any unusual signs. Return pack to unit and dispose of towels. Proceed with therapeutic exercise. Approximately 20 min is required to reheat the hydrocollator packs after each use (see figure 5.1).

■ **Figure 5.1** Hot pack: adequate toweling must be used. Heat therapy is more helpful when combined with passive or active range of motion.

PARAFFIN

Paraffin wax has a melting point of 130° F but remains in a liquid form at 118 to 130° F when mixed with mineral oil. The paraffin mixture has a low specific heat (the number of calories required to raise 1 g of the substance 1° C). This means that the body is able to tolerate higher temperatures of the paraffin mixture without scalding.

Paraffin is a superficial heat modality used most commonly with the hand, wrist, foot, and ankle. The mineral oil leaves the skin soft and slightly oily—a good premassage condition. Furthermore, the modality provides circumferential heating and allows elevation.

To apply paraffin, first check the temperature of the paraffin bath. The treatment temperature should range from 118 to 130° F (depending on the mixture of wax/ mineral oil). Inspect the area to be treated. Open lesions or new scars should not be submersed in paraffin. The treatment area should be thoroughly washed and dried, and all jewelry should be removed. Explain the treatment to the athlete. The wax may feel hot at first, but it should not burn. You may have to demonstrate with a finger.

Using the hand as an example, we will describe the "dip and wrap" and "dip and reimmerse" techniques. For the dip and wrap technique, spread the fingers and dip the hand into the tank. Remove the hand immediately. Do not move the fingers or the hand after the initial dip. Allow the dripping to stop before dipping the hand again. After six to eight dips, wrap the hand with a plastic bag and then in a towel. Elevate the hand above the heart for 15 to 20 min.

For the dip and reimmerse technique, follow the preceding instructions, but after eight dips, immerse the hand in the paraffin bath for 15 to 20 min. This is a more vigorous heating technique but requires the hand to be in a dependent position throughout the treatment. After treatment, remove the wax "glove" and return wax to the tank. Wipe perspiration and excess oil from the hand. The mineral oil often prepares the treatment area for massage (see figure 5.2).

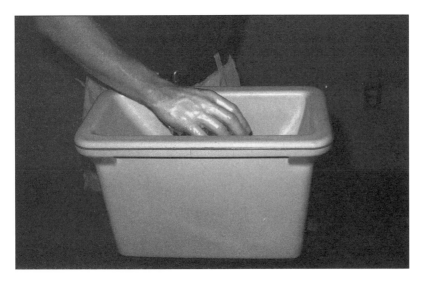

∎ Figure 5.2   Paraffin wax. Temperature of the mixture should be within 118° to 130° F. The hand should be in a comfortable, relaxed position. Dip into the wax and let it drip. Continue to add layers of wax by re-dipping, and then either wrap in plastic or submerge into the wax for an additional 15 to 20 min.

FLUIDOTHERAPY

Fluidotherapy is a dry heating agent. Cellulose particles (corncob flakes) are suspended through forced air. Therefore, this modality shares features of hydrotherapy, although it is dry heat convection. The particles create a resistance, so active exercise is possible. Manufacturers claim that the particles are self-sterilizing so the unit requires minimal care. This modality is most commonly used in treating hand injuries but can be adapted for other body parts. The recommended treatment temperature ranges from 110 to 125° F, which does not burn because the hot air is less able to create thermal changes than water is.

To apply fluidotherapy, have the athlete wash and dry the body part thoroughly. Protect any open lesion by using a loose rubber glove or a plastic bag. Warm the unit to the desired temperature and activate the unit by turning on the timer. Position the athlete comfortably. Insert the extremity and secure the Velcro straps. Make sure the athlete does not remove the straps during the treatment or the particles will spill from the machine. Set the timer for 15 to 20 min and adjust the agitation. As more air is forced through the particles, the resistance decreases (see figure 5.3).

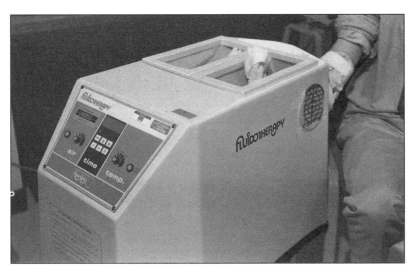

∎ Figure 5.3
Fluidotherapy unit.

HYDROTHERAPY

Hydrotherapy allows complete heating of the involved body part, and active exercise or range of motion can be performed simultaneously with the heat therapy. Additionally, the agitation can act as a counterirritant to reduce pain. However, because the body cannot dissipate the heat as well, care should be taken to avoid overheating when most of the body is submerged. When whirlpool treatments are used, the water temperature may range from 37 to 45° C (98-110° F), depending on the amount of surface area submerged. The body has less ability to cool itself when

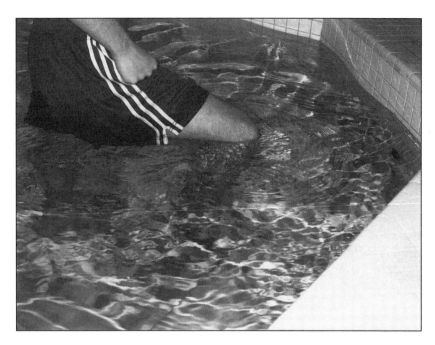

■ Figure 5.4 Hydrotherapy (warm whirlpool) allows active range of motion during the heat treatment.

large areas are heated, so lower temperatures should be used with jacuzzi or whole-body submersion. In a jacuzzi or whole-body submersion, the blood pressure is lowered and the heart rate increases to dissipate the heat, so any person with a cardiovascular history should be monitored closely and should be limited to 10 min in the pool. Tanks must be cleaned after use to prevent cross-contamination if a filtration system is not available (see figure 5.4).

CONTRAST THERAPY

Contrast therapy takes advantage of the benefits of heat (decreased pain and increased range of motion) while limiting the inflammatory reaction of the increased temperature. Some clinicians propose that contrast therapy reduces edema because of the vasodilation and vasoconstriction of the prearteriole sphincters; however, this has not been documented. It is likely that the exposure to either the heat or cold is not long enough to cause any measurable reaction. The benefit of contrast therapy lies in the sensory overload, which can decrease pain. This pain reduction can promote range of motion when exercise is done simultaneously with the submersion. The treatment generally alternates between hot and cold, often ending in cold because therapeutic exercise is usually the next procedure (see figure 5.5). Contrast is empirically helpful in warming up the ankle joint to increase motion before exercise after swelling has stabilized.

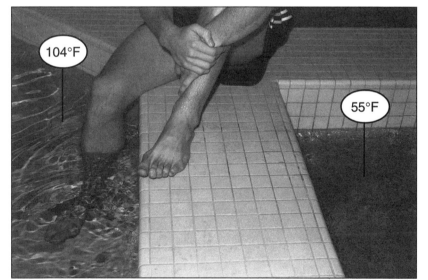

104°F

55°F

■ Figure 5.5 Contrast whirlpool. Subacute: 2 min hot (AROM), 2 min cold; shows tolerance to heat: 3 min hot (AROM), 2 min cold; warm-up for exercise: 4 min hot (AROM), 1 min cold.

CRITERIA FOR MOVING FROM COLD TO HEAT

Most emergency rooms or physicians instruct their patients to use heat on a musculoskeletal injury for 48 h after the injury occurs. Although this may be appropriate for some people who limit their activity, it is not acceptable practice when an athletic trainer is available to monitor progress and begin therapeutic exercise. The athletic trainer should systematically evaluate the injury to determine when or if heat is an appropriate treatment, because acute inflammation may last longer than 48 h and it would be contraindicated to use heat during this time. Additionally, exercise or activity may cause an inflammatory reaction, in which case ice should remain the treatment of choice (see figure 5.6).

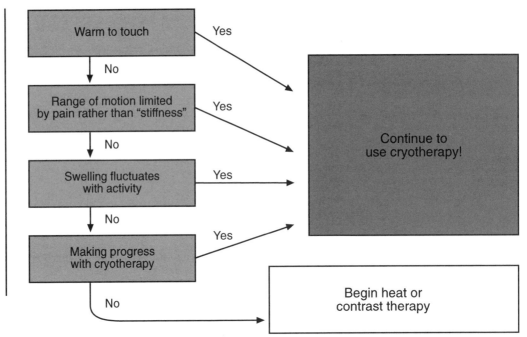

▌Figure 5.6 Criteria for moving from cold treatments to heat.

INDICATIONS AND CONTRAINDICATIONS FOR SUPERFICIAL HEAT

Superficial heat can be used for the following conditions:

- Joint or connective tissue stiffness (restricted range of motion)
- Muscle spasm
- Pain
- Conditions in which superficial blood flow is desired

Superficial heat should not be used with the following conditions:

- Decreased sensation (the patient cannot perceive the heat, and burns may result)
- Decreased circulation (as occurs with diabetes or cardiac conditions, which result in an inability to dissipate the heat by increasing blood flow)
- Inflammatory conditions
- Presence of cancers or neoplasms

Name_____ Date_____

Activities

1. Set up a volunteer with the various types of superficial heat: hot packs, paraffin bath, hot whirlpool, or fluidotherapy. Note the benefits and disadvantages of each method of heat application.

2. In the following patient problems, demonstrate, discuss, and note the type of superficial heat used, the position of the patient, and the length of the treatment:
   * Hamstring "tightness"
   * Decreased range of motion of the ankle
   * Flexion contracture of the proximal interphalangeal joint of the middle finger
   * Low back pain and spasm
   * Delayed onset muscle soreness in the gluts, quads, and hamstrings
   * Shoulder stiffness

3. Use the following case studies to discuss and note the clinical use of heat and cold. There are no "right" answers because of the individual interpretation of the scenarios. Justify what modality you would use based on the effects of superficial heat and cold.

   Case A: An athlete has subacute subacromial bursitis in the left shoulder. There is decreased glenohumeral motion due to pain.

   Case B: An athlete sustained a quadriceps strain 4 days ago and now has weakness and stiffness in this muscle. The area is not warm to touch or red.

Case C: A soccer player sprained his ankle 24 h ago. There is minimal effusion or edema, but the ankle is painful, especially with motion. Explain the treatment.

Would your method change if there was significant edema present? If so, how?

Case D: A field hockey player complains of "shin splints" on the right leg with a tender area approximately 4 + 4 cm medial to the tibia.

Case E: You determine that a basketball player has sustained an acute knee contusion and is unable to walk without a limp. You notice that there is a hematoma forming on the prepatellar area.

Case F: A wrestler complains of pain and spasm of the upper trap. You can palpate localized areas of pain trigger points.

4. Assess a partner's hamstring flexibility. One group of students applies heat and stretch, whereas one group applies heat only. Remeasure hamstring flexibility, and note your results in the table below.

Pretest	Posttest	+15 min	+30 min

LAB 6

Principles of Electrotherapy

Review material from chapter 8, pages 124 to 131 of the textbook, before you complete this lab.

OBJECTIVES

- You will be able to identify various waveforms and identify the components of the waveform.

- You will be able to determine the polarity of different types of electrical stimulators and which features are characteristic of that particular type of machine.

- You will understand the relationship between the amplitude and phase duration of the waveform.

- You will understand how the pulse frequency affects the perception of electrical stimulation.

MONOPHASIC AND BIPHASIC WAVEFORMS

To understand the different types of electrical stimulators available, it is important to discuss the characteristics of the current applied to the body. The waveform describes the configuration of pulses of the electrical current. Very strict definitions have been assigned to waveforms such as alternating current (AC) and direct current (DC) to provide consistent terminology within physical medicine and to minimize confusion when communicating with other professions. There are two major classifications of waveforms: monophasic and biphasic. DC and AC can be categorized as monophasic and biphasic, respectively, but DC and AC have no interruption between each pulse and continue indefinitely. Monophasic currents have uniquely positive and negative electrodes, whereas biphasic currents shift polarity continually and each electrode has identical effects if the waveform is symmetrical. Polar effects to the tissues are minimized or eliminated with a biphasic current (see figure 6.1).

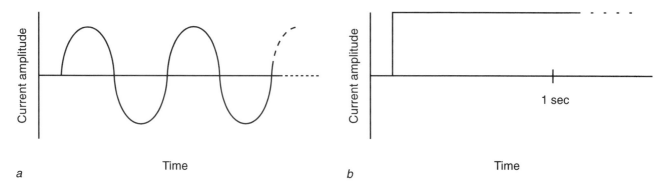

■ **Figure 6.1**   Continuous currents. *(a)* Alternating current (AC): continuous sinusoidal, biphasic current with no interruption between each pulse. There is an inverse relationship between the phase duration and pulse frequency. *(b)* Direct current (DC): monophasic current that flows in one direction for longer than one second.

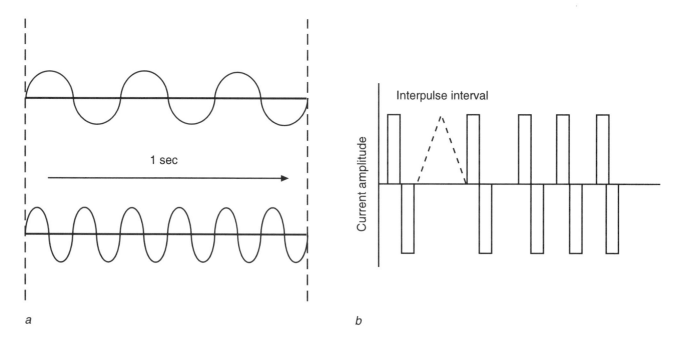

■ **Figure 6.2**   Relationship of frequency to pulse duration. *(a)* Alternating current has no interruptions between pulses and has an inverse relationship of pulse duration to frequency. *(b)* A pulsatile current has interruptions called interpulse intervals between each pulse that eliminate the relationship between pulse duration and frequency.

Modulation of the waveform within the unit produces pulsatile currents, which have temporary interruptions between each pulse. Pulsatile currents have various shapes, phase durations (usually short), and interpulse spacings. The space between each pulse eliminates the normal inverse relationship between frequency and wavelength as with AC. This allows the clinician to independently control the number of pulses per second (frequency) and the phase duration of pulsatile currents (see figures 6.2 and 6.3).

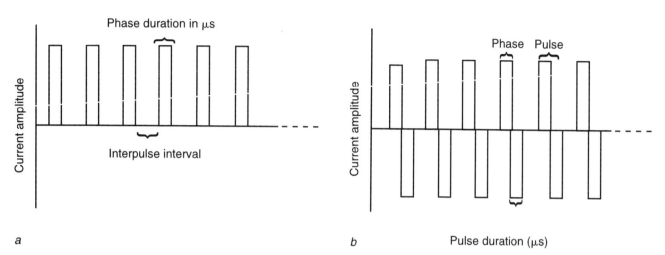

a   b   Pulse duration (μs)

■ **Figure 6.3**   Pulsatile monophasic and biphasic currents. *(a)* Monophasic current flows in one direction only. One electrode is always positive (+) and the other is always negative (−). The interpulse interval allows independent control of phase duration and pulse frequency. *(b)* Pulsatile biphasic current flows in one direction, then the other. Neither electrode is positive (+) or negative (−) since they constantly switch. Each pulse (two phases) is separated by an interpulse interval, and there is independent control of pulse duration and frequency.

PARAMETERS OF THE ELECTRICAL STIMULATION

The parameters that need to be considered and are often manipulated by the clinician are phase duration, amplitude, and pulse frequency.

PHASE DURATION AND AMPLITUDE

Phase duration is the time to complete one phase of a pulse and affects the type of fiber recruited. Amplitude refers to the intensity or magnitude of the current. The peak current is the maximum amplitude of the current at any point during the pulse without regard to its duration. A high peak current has a greater depth of penetration, which allows more fibers to be recruited (figure 6.4). Average current, however, refers to the amount of current supplied over a period of time, which takes into consideration both the peak amplitude and the phase duration. Depending on the waveform, it is possible to have a high peak but low average current, which is a characteristic of a high-voltage stimulator. The average current ultimately determines the physiochemical response of a tissue and, if too high, can damage tissue. Often, the average current is lowered to a safer level by modifying the waveform or parameters, specifically the phase duration (see figure 6.5).

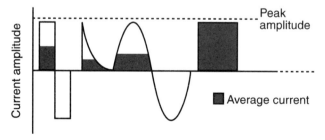

■ **Figure 6.4**   Peak amplitude and average current.

The phase duration and amplitude are related when you are determining whether a specific nerve fiber can be targeted by using the parameters available on an electri-

Phase duration

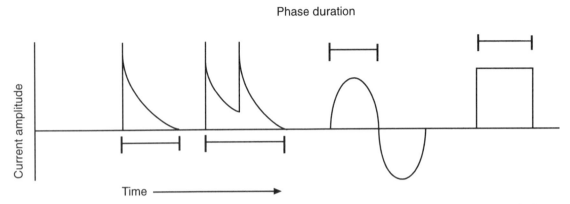

■ **Figure 6.5**   Phase duration: length of time current flows in one direction before turning off or switching polarity.

cal stimulator. Because of the capacitance of each nerve fiber type, a limiting phase duration must be exceeded to cause an action potential. However, when a waveform has a long phase duration, small increases in amplitude cause a stronger sensory or motor reaction. The relationship between the amplitude and phase duration is called the strength–duration curve (see figure 6.6).

Each tissue type has a specific strength–duration curve depending on the capacitance of the tissue and the depth of the target tissue. The A-beta (large diameter, sensory nerve) has the lowest capacitance and is therefore the most easily simulated. The A-beta, A-alpha (motor nerve), and A-delta (large diameter, pain fibers) are stimulated in the microsecond phase duration range (10^{-6}), which is common with most TENS units. C fibers and muscle tissue have much greater capacitance and require stimulation in the millisecond range (10^{-3}) (see figure 6.7).

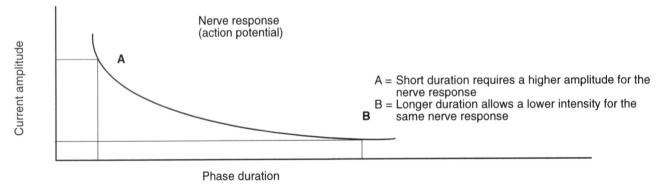

■ **Figure 6.6**   Strength–duration curve.

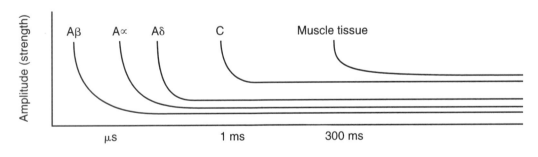

■ **Figure 6.7**   Strength–duration curves for various tissues. Because of the capacitance of the tissues, sensory nerves are the most easily excitable and can reach an action potential with a short phase duration. C fibers and the muscle membrane are difficult to excite and require much longer phase durations.

FREQUENCY

The frequency of the stimulation is the number of pulses generated per second (pps or hertz). The frequency affects the number of action potentials elicited during the stimulation. Although the same number of fibers are recruited, a higher frequency causes them to fire at a more rapid pace, which ultimately increases the tension generated. Nerve membranes must repolarize, however, after discharging. There is an absolute refractory period in which the resting membrane potential is reinstated, and another action potential cannot be elicited during this time. The absolute refractory period is ultimately the rate-limiting factor of the number of impulses that can be generated by a nerve.

The rate of rise of the leading edge of the pulse is a parameter that is incorporated into a waveform, but it also will affect the type of nerve targeted. The rate of rise is the time it takes to get from zero to maximal amplitude within each pulse. Fast rates of rise times are necessary, especially with low-capacitance tissues such as large motor nerves. The low-capacitance membrane cannot store charge and quickly accommodates to a stimulus. These nerves can dissipate the charge from a pulse with slow rates of rise times, and the ion flux needed to alter the voltage to exceed threshold is never reached. Sensory nerves that carry light touch, for example, have low capacitance and easily accommodate. This explains how a person is aware of clothing when it is first put on, but there is accommodation to this minimal stimulus and the person no longer pays attention to the sensation at the skin. Generally, tissues with low capacitance accommodate to a stimulus easily, whereas high-capacitance tissues, because they store the charge, do not accommodate or dissipate the charge readily.

When determining whether there will be a physiological response within the tissues, three important factors within each pulse of an electrical current must be considered. First, the stimulus must be of adequate amplitude to reach the threshold level of excitatory tissues. Second, the rate of voltage change (rate of rise of the leading edge of the pulse) must be rapid enough that tissue accommodation cannot take place. Third, the length of stimulus or phase duration must be long enough to overcome the capacitance of the tissue to allow an action potential.

DUTY CYCLE

The final parameter of electrical stimulation is the duty cycle. Duty cycles can be imposed by the clinician to interrupt the current periodically for several seconds. This on/off time creates a rest time that is variable on most units. Pulses also can be incorporated into duty cycles inherently in the machine, which creates envelopes or packages of pulses. These duty cycles interrupt the current at specific intervals so that the manufacturer can produce "time modulated AC" currents, otherwise known as "burst mode." The carrier frequency is usually an AC and is interrupted at regular intervals, often in the millisecond range. Interruptions are generally imperceptible but they enable the clinician to take advantage of the characteristics of the carrier frequency. The classical Russian stimulators use this method to modulate medium-frequency sinusoidal waves into bursts of 10 ms on and 10 ms off. The duty cycle also manipulates medium frequency generators to physiologically active frequencies, which are less than 1000 Hz (figure 6.8).

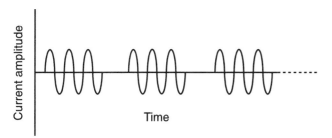

Figure 6.8 Phase duration.

Name_____ Date_____

Activities

1. Practice drawing the different types of waveforms: 1) biphasic square wave, 2) sinusoidal (AC), 3) direct current, 4) twin peak monophasic, 5) asymmetrical biphasic wave, 6) time-modulated AC with carrier frequency of 1000 Hz modulated to five bursts per second. Label the (a) amplitude, (b) phase duration, (c) pulse duration if applicable, and (d) interpulse interval. Draw at least three cycles of each.

Biphasic square wave

_____

Sinusoidal (AC)

_____

Direct current

_____

Twin peak monophasic

_____

Asymmetrical biphasic wave

_____

Time-modulated AC with carrier frequency of 1000 Hz modulated to five bursts per second

_____

2. Apply an electrical stimulator and determine the minimal intensity needed to cause a muscle contraction when the phase duration is 50 μs. Plot the intensities needed to cause a minimal contraction when the phase duration is 75, 100, 125, 150, 175, and 200 μs.

Intensity (amplitude)

75	100	125	150	175	200

Time (μs)

3. Determine what pulse rate is necessary to cause a strong, even contraction (called *tetany*). Starting at a low frequency (< 5 pps), increase the pulse rate. Note below at what frequency the individual pulses are no longer perceptible and what else happens to the perception of the electricity.

- 5 pps
- 10 pps
- 15 pps
- 20 pps
- 25 pps

- 30 pps
- 35 pps
- 40 pps
- 45 pps
- 50 pps

4. For a 1-sec time interval, draw a symmetrical biphasic current that has 3 pps, 150 μs phase duration, and 100 mA amplitude. What happens to the total current when the rate is increased to 5 pps? What happens when the phase duration is increased to 200 μs, and what happens when the amplitude is increased to 150 mA? What is expected to happen to the perception of the current as these parameters change?

_____

_____

_____

LAB 7

Electrode Considerations

This material is not covered in the textbook.

OBJECTIVES

- You will be able to recognize various types of electrodes that are used with electrotherapy.

- You will understand how to reduce resistance within electrodes.

- You will understand current density with respect to electrodes.

- You will understand monopolar and bipolar electrode configurations.

- You will be able to choose an appropriate electrode configuration.

TYPES OF ELECTRODES

To complete a circuit in electrical stimulation, at least one electrode from each output lead must be in contact with the athlete's skin (see figure 7.1). There will always be resistance to the current from the air–skin interface, and to increase efficiency and consistency of the treatment, the clinician should minimize the resistance.

Many types of electrodes are available for electrical stimulation. Portable TENS units often use "single-use" or disposable electrodes that are self-adhesive. These electrodes are convenient, minimize the irritation of the skin that often occurs with tape adherents, and make the application simple. The electrodes may be remoistened with water when moved to a new location. The expense of these electrodes may prohibit their use when there is heavy volume.

Most electrodes for commercial or clinical use are either metal-backed or carbon rubber. These require an interface such as moistened sponges or gauze. Gel may be used with the carbon rubber electrodes; however, this may reduce the longevity of the electrodes if they are not cleaned properly. Sponges are the most convenient, but gauze is more sanitary. The interface should be thoroughly wet with no dry spots, but not dripping.

Minimizing Electrode Resistance

- Use large electrodes
- Maintain even, firm contact with skin
- Use clean electrodes and sponges
- Keep the sponge interface well moistened
- Remove excess hair and oil from skin

The electrodes should be attached firmly to the athlete by using elastic straps. Weights may be used to secure the electrodes to the low back; however, the current density will change drastically if the electrodes move or become displaced during the treatment. This may cause discomfort to the athlete. The intensity should be adjusted after the electrodes have been secured because any adjustment in the air–skin interface will affect the resistance and potentially can increase the amplitude

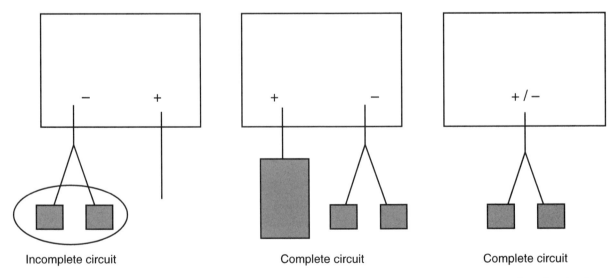

Incomplete circuit   Complete circuit   Complete circuit

∎ **Figure 7.1** Monophasic versus biphasic stimulators. Make sure there are at least two leads to complete the circuit to allow stimulation. The electrode configuration on the left does not complete the circuit.

dramatically. Electrodes should be flexible to conform to body parts such as the ankle or knee.

Any lead can be bifurcated, or divided. It is imperative that each lead be used because a common mistake in applying electrical stimulation is to use one bifurcated lead (two electrodes), which does not complete the circuit and therefore delivers no stimulation. Whenever bifurcated leads are used, current density becomes an issue. Each lead may be bifurcated as many times as needed.

UNDERSTANDING CURRENT DENSITY

Current density depends on the size of the electrodes and their distance apart. There will be an equal amount of current in each of the two essential leads. When unequal-sized electrodes are used, the current is more concentrated in the smaller electrode. This causes a perception of increased intensity under the smaller electrode. When electrodes are very different in size, such as with a point stimulator, the patient may not be able to perceive current in the larger electrode. The larger electrode becomes the dispersive electrode because the current is dispersed over a broad area. When bifurcating leads, it is important to determine the total size of all electrodes that arise from each lead and compare that total to the opposite lead (see figure 7.2).

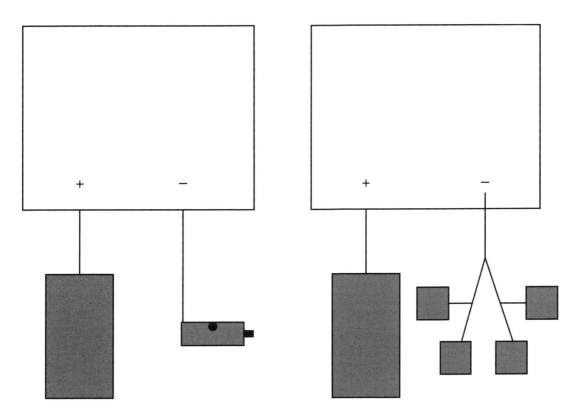

■ Figure 7.2   Current density concentrates current in the lead that has the smallest total surface area.

Current density also can refer to the concentration of current within the tissues. Current always flows in the path of least resistance. If the electrodes are placed very close together, the current is most dense or concentrated in the superficial tissues. If the electrodes are distant to each other, then the current has the potential to take a deeper path through the nerve and blood vessels that have less resistance.

DETERMINING POLARITY

All stimulators use either a monophasic or biphasic current. You can determine the polarity by examining the stimulator. If the stimulator has a polarity switch, then the stimulator is monophasic and the toggle will determine the polarity of the active lead. The active lead is demarcated on the unit as well. Additionally, most monophasic machines have leads that arise from different locations on the stimulator, whereas most biphasic units have the two essential leads arising from the same location or socket from the stimulator. In a biphasic machine, there is no physiological difference between the electrodes, and therefore it is not necessary to distinguish the leads (figure 7.3).

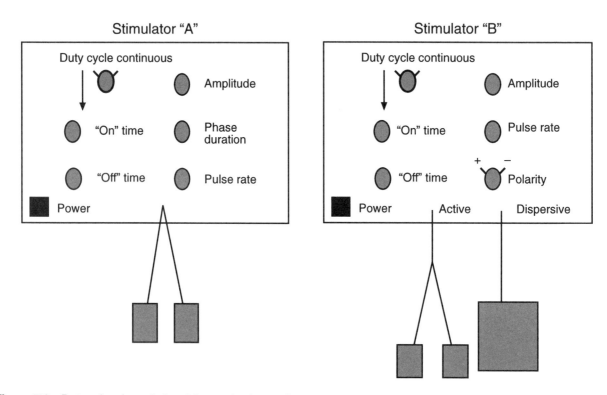

■ **Figure 7.3**   Determine the polarity of these stimulators. Stimulator A has no polarity switch and both leads arise from the same location. Stimulator B has a polarity switch and each lead is distinct.

ELECTRODE CONFIGURATIONS

The most common types of electrode configurations are monopolar, bipolar, and quadripolar. Either monopolar or bipolar may be used with monophasic or biphasic currents. Quadripolar electrode configurations are often used with interferential current.

MONOPOLAR ELECTRODE CONFIGURATION

With a monopolar electrode configuration, two or more unequal-sized electrodes are used. One lead is designated as "active" and the other is designated as "dispersive." The leads are placed at different locations, with the active lead placed at target site and the dispersive lead placed away from the treatment site. There are three primary reasons for using a monopolar electrode configuration. One is to place the electrodes farther apart so there is deeper penetration. An example would be with underwater stimulation, where there is less resistance in the water so the current preferentially would go through the water instead of though the skin. When a monopolar configuration is used, the current has to travel through the body to reach the other electrode, which is at a distant site to the treatment location. The second reason for using a monopolar electrode configuration is to counter the intensity at the pointed end of a point stimulator. The small electrode with a high current density is desired at the treatment site, but it is more comfortable to use a larger electrode to complete the circuit. Often the patient does not perceive current under the larger electrode. Finally, a monopolar electrode configuration is required when a polarity effect is desired. A monophasic current must be used to differentiate the polarity at the treatment site from the other lead. The polarity is indicated by the active lead. Examples of this method are iontophoresis or when creating an electrical field of a particular polarity, such as with wound healing (see figure 7.4).

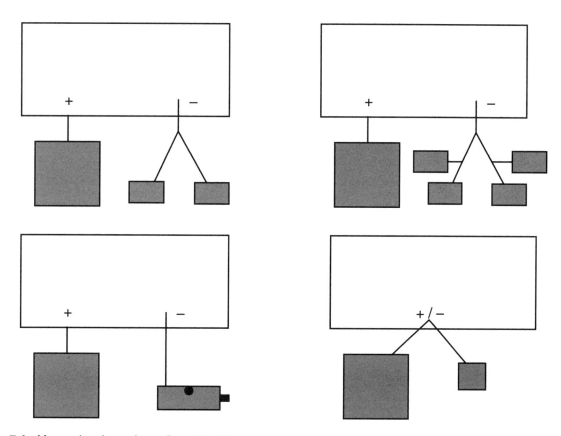

Figure 7.4 Monopolar electrode configuration. Note that either a monophasic or biphasic machine can be used. Each example uses different-sized electrodes.

BIPOLAR ELECTRODE CONFIGURATION

Bipolar electrode configurations also can be used with either monophasic or biphasic currents. In this case, equal-sized electrodes are used, with both placed over the treatment site. This setup is the most commonly used method in TENS (see figure 7.5).

QUADRIPOLAR ELECTRODE CONFIGURATION

This type of electrode configuration is often used with interferential current. Two completely separate, medium-frequency generators are used, and the electrodes are placed to cross the currents. Ideally, the current is *interfered* (see lab 11) in the center

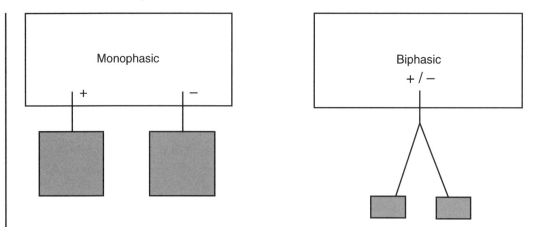

■ **Figure 7.5** Bipolar electrode configuration. Similar-sized electrodes are used with either a monophasic or biphasic machine.

of the two currents; however, because the body is not homogeneous, the current may vary. Many interferential stimulators have an adjustment that allows variation in the amplitude of one of the currents so that the location of the perceived current can be adjusted.

Quadripolar electrode configuration is not the same as using two channels of TENS with four electrodes. Using two channels with TENS increases the number of stimulation points, which may be advantageous when treating a large surface area; however, the currents do not cross and cause interference (see figure 7.6).

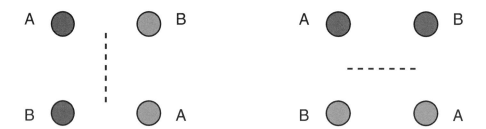

■ **Figure 7.6** Quadripolar electrode configuration used with interferential current. The current is aligned so that it is concentrated between the electrodes to localize the stimulation depending on the pathology. A and B are the two channels.

Name_____ Date_____

Activities

1. Examine the electrical stimulators available in the lab or the athletic training room. Determine and note below the waveform of each unit.

2. Examine various types of electrodes. Use different methods of applying these electrodes and determine the best way to minimize the skin–electrode resistance. Note below which types of electrodes require additional care.

3. Set up both monophasic and biphasic units with either monopolar or bipolar electrode configurations. Which types of machines lend themselves most easily to each? When would each be most advantageous? List three situations in which you would use each machine.

4. Bifurcate the leads, if possible, by using a monopolar electrode configuration. Determine whether there is perception in the dispersive electrode. Note below what happens to the current density when the leads are bifurcated.

LAB 8

Transcutaneous Electrical Nerve Stimulation for Pain

Review material from chapter 8, pages 136 to 146 of the textbook, before you complete this lab.

OBJECTIVES

- You will be able to apply the different pain theories with TENS parameters.

- You will be able to determine the best electrical stimulator and parameters to treat various painful conditions.

- You will understand how the site of electrode application affects the treatment.

- You will understand when the athlete requires a TENS unit and establish a protocol for explaining the application to the athlete.

TRANSCUTANEOUS ELECTRICAL NERVE STIMULATION (TENS)

Pain modulation is the primary reason for TENS. Review the pain-modulation theories presented earlier, because the techniques described in this lab will follow those theories.

TENS units are often versatile in their parameters and often allow the clinician freedom to manipulate the phase duration, frequency, amplitude, and duty cycle. Examples of TENS units include high-voltage stimulators, interferential units, microcurrent, and some low-voltage stimulators. Although any type of electrical stimulator that crosses the skin to excite the nerve is considered to be TENS, there are other uses of these stimulators including edema reduction, wound healing, and muscle stimulation.

Variations of TENS can be achieved by adjusting the current parameters. The proposed mechanisms of pain modulation appropriate for each type of electrical stimulation will be discussed. Because therapy with electrical stimulation treats the symptoms of an ailment and generally not the cause, proper evaluation of the etiology of the injury and rectification of the cause are important. Ideally, the pain modulation allows the athlete to perform therapeutic exercise, which will help alleviate the problem.

Do not use electrical stimulation if there are known myocardial problems or arrhythmias. TENS should not be used if there is a pacemaker or if pregnancy is suspected. Electrical stimulation should not be delivered through the chest or over the carotid sinus. Stimulation in the anterior neck elicits activity in the carotid sinus or may cause a contraction of the pharyngeal muscles, which can affect the blood pressure and pulse.

SENSORY TENS

Sensory TENS is also called *high-rate TENS* and can be used for any painful condition, most commonly in the acute phase or postoperatively. The submotor stimulation is comfortable, providing excitation of large afferent (sensory) nerves. Pain reduction is attributed to the spinal gate mechanism. The duration of pain relief generally lasts only as long as the stimulation. Any machine that allows stimulation of large-diameter sensory nerves can be used for this treatment. Sensory TENS commonly is used to reduce pain after an injury or after surgery in combination with ice, elevation, and compression.

To apply sensory TENS, the following parameters should be available on the unit: phase duration, pulse rate, and amplitude. The target nerve fiber is A-beta (sensory), which has a low capacitance and therefore does not require a very long phase duration. The phase duration should be low and generally is less than 100 µs. Longer phase durations increase the possibility of stimulating pain fibers, which should be avoided in sensory TENS. The pulse rate should be set high, generally 60 to 120 pps. The pulse rate should be high enough that the athlete cannot differentiate the individual pulses. The amplitude should create a strong sensory perception but remain submotor. If the muscles begin to contract, lower the amplitude. There should not be a duty cycle with this type of treatment, and the stimulator should be set in the continuous mode.

The treatment time theoretically can last up to 24 h. However, the athlete can be instructed to use the device for intermittent 20- to 30-min treatments to see whether the pain diminishes. If pain is not reduced, then electrode placement should be adjusted. Emphasize that TENS treatments do not replace other aspects of rehabilitation, such as exercise. The electrical stimulation often relieves symptoms but does not address the pathology as therapeutic exercise does. When used in the athletic training room, TENS treatments generally are combined with ice or heat to reduce pain or spasm. The treatment time is based on which therapies are used, ranging

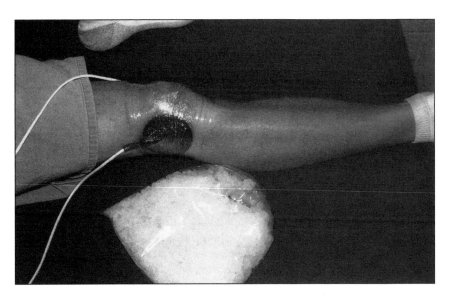

from 10 to 45 min depending on the depth of the target structure for the heat or cold therapy (see figure 8.1).

MOTOR TENS

Motor TENS may also be referred to as *low-rate TENS* and has been equated with acupuncture in its mechanism of pain relief. This mode of TENS is based on the motor pain modulation theory. Motor TENS is more vigorous than sensory TENS and is used to treat subacute pain or trigger points. Motor TENS should not be used on acute injuries where vigorous contrac-

■ Figure 8.1 Sensory TENS is often used with ice as a pain management technique with acute injuries. Make sure the electrodes do not insulate the area so that effective cooling may take place.

tions may increase discomfort or cause bleeding.

Motor stimulation is theorized to release endogenous opiates and may provide relief for a longer duration, lasting from 1 to 3 h after a 30-min treatment. Pain relief may be delayed compared with sensory TENS but lasts for a longer duration, sometimes as long as 4 h.

To apply motor TENS, set the phase duration, pulse rate, and amplitude to the following specifications. The phase duration should be high, in a range of 200 to 300 μs to target the A-delta (fast pain) nerve fiber. Because the motor nerve fibers are deep, elicitation of the A-delta fibers corresponds to a visible muscle contraction. The pulse rate should be low with distinct, separate pulses in the range of 2 to 4 pps. The amplitude should elicit strong, visible contractions but should not cause pain. A strong, tolerable muscle contraction indicates the stimulation of A-delta fibers. Treatment time generally lasts 20 to 30 min, although the pain relief may not occur for 30 to 120 min. A duty cycle is not necessary for motor TENS, and the continuous mode should be selected.

It is sometimes recommended that treatment be initiated with the sensory TENS technique to relieve pain quickly. As the pain subsides, the parameters can be adjusted to deliver motor TENS for prolonged pain relief. Again, this should be used only when the muscle contractions do not cause injury.

NOXIOUS TENS

A noxious stimulus is applied to relieve pain through the central biasing mechanism. This mode of TENS commonly is used with point stimulators because the amplitude should be the maximum tolerable level to trigger descending serotonergic tracts to inhibit pain. The small diameter of the probe creates a high current density to the target area without subjecting a broad area to the noxious stimulus. Units may incorporate an ohmmeter to identify points of lower skin resistance that correlate highly with trigger and acupuncture points. Body charts may help locate appropriate points for optimal pain relief.

The key to appropriate noxious TENS is to use a machine that allows the stimulation of C fibers. Very few machines allow a phase duration long enough to elicit a response of C fibers because long phase durations have the potential to apply a great deal of current. The Neuroprobe or a galvanic stimulator can be used. The phase duration should be greater than 10 to 20 ms. This is in contrast with most TENS units, which have a maximum of 250 μs (milli [m] = 10^{-3}; micro [μ] = 10^{-6}).

To apply noxious TENS, the parameters should be set to the following specifications. Again, the ability to stimulate C fibers may be prohibited in many stimulators to protect the athlete. The phase duration should be longer than 1 ms and the amplitude should be as high as tolerable. The pulse rate may vary, but you should choose either a high frequency or low frequency. The high-frequency 100 to 150 pps prevents the discrimination of individual pulses and is classically used in noxious TENS. A low frequency of 2 to 7 pps, however, will elicit the benefits of motor TENS in conjunction with noxious TENS. If the stimulator parameters are capable of overcoming the capacitance C fibers, then the A-delta fibers will be stimulated as well, providing an added benefit. Each point should be stimulated for 30 sec, and generally 8 to 10 points are treated in a session.

Do not expect good results for TENS treatments if the athlete is taking narcotic analgesics. The electrical stimulation produces natural opiates that compete for the receptor sites that are occupied by the medication. See table 8.1 for a comparison of different types of TENS.

Table 8.1   TENS Parameters

Type of TENS	Phase duration	Pulse frequency	Amplitude	Target nerve fiber
Sensory	< 100 μs	60-120 pps	Sensory, submotor	Aβ
Motor	200–300 μs	2-4 pps	Strong contractions	Aδ
Noxious	> 1 ms	2-4 pps or 100-150 pps	Tolerable pain	C fiber

POINT STIMULATION

The following procedure describes the location of acupuncture or trigger points with the Neuroprobe or ohmmeter. Refer to body or acupuncture charts and determine appropriate landmarks. Explain the procedure to the athlete, who should hold the dispersive electrode. Calibrate the sensitivity of the unit by applying the probe to the skin to determine the baseline skin resistance. Dead skin or oils reduce conductivity and make the location of points more difficult. With even pressure, move the probe along the skin over the site of the trigger point. An auditory signal or a large change in skin resistance signal identifies the location of the point (see figure 8.2).

For point stimulation, follow the procedure for point location, and then start increasing the amplitude. Make sure to reset the intensity to zero after each point. Increase the intensity until the athlete reports the perception of sensation. Because the current may change the skin impedance, a breakthrough phenomenon

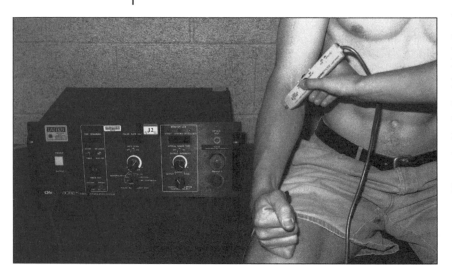

▮ **Figure 8.2** Neuroprobe point stimulation. A monopolar electrode configuration is used with the active electrode in the remote and the dispersive electrode in the athlete's hand.

may occur. The intensity may seem to be increased suddenly to an intolerable level. You must be able to rapidly adjust the amplitude during the stimulation to maintain a maximum but tolerable noxious output. Stimulate each point for 30 sec. Repeat the treatment on each point two to three times or until the noxious intensity is sustained for at least 20 sec.

Work from distal to proximal, and treat 8 to 12 points at each treatment. Inspect the skin after the treatment. Micropunctate burns can result from this treatment but are inconsequential and resolve. This treatment should be done no more than once per day to take advantage of the endogenous opiate production (too frequent stimulation causes a less dramatic pain relief).

PORTABLE TENS UNITS

Battery-operated portable TENS units allow a long duration of electrical stimulation. They can be loaned or sold to an athlete or patient so that TENS can be used throughout the day or night for pain management. Portable TENS units often are used for electrical stimulation treatments when the athlete is traveling with a team. The athlete should be taught to use the stimulator if portable TENS treatments are to continue. The athletic trainer must educate the athlete about how to use the unit, when to use the stimulator, where to place the electrodes, and how to care for the skin.

When an athlete uses a portable TENS unit, the athletic trainer completes a musculoskeletal evaluation to determine the source of pain and areas of associated pain. From the evaluation, determine sites for electrode placement, which may be around a painful joint, on trigger or acupuncture points, at spinal nerve root levels or peripheral nerve trunks, or at a superficial point of the nerve supplying the painful area. The athletic trainer should prepare the skin site by cleaning the area; electrodes should not be placed over abraded skin or open wounds. Secure electrodes at designated areas on the skin. Carbon-silicon-impregnated rubber electrodes require a conductive gel interface. Some pregelled electrodes contain an adherent. Thoroughly explain the treatment to the athlete.

Preset the phase duration and the pulse rate before application according to the type of TENS to be used. Gradually increase the amplitude until the athlete feels a tingling sensation. Increase the amplitude until the stimulation is strong but comfortable. Electrodes may have to be adjusted for better stimulation and pain relief. The athlete can be taught to adjust the amplitude independently but to keep the stimulation at the desired intensity (motor or submotor).

During treatment, the amplitude may be adjusted to maximize pain relief and to account for accommodation. The fast response to sensory TENS allows rapid evaluation of electrode placement and effectiveness. If the athlete responds beneficially to sensory TENS, you can use other modes. After 20 to 30 min, reevaluate the athlete for pain and inspect electrode sites for hyperemia.

The athlete may be instructed in home use. Sensory TENS can be used throughout the day, but the athlete should be taught to turn the stimulation off periodically and monitor the duration of pain relief (figure 8.3).

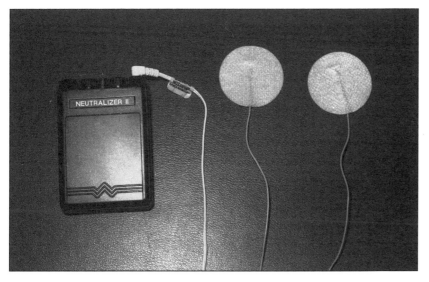

Figure 8.3 Portable TENS units are available from many manufacturers. Most have two channels and allow the clinician to preadjust the rate, phase duration, and modulation.

MODULATION MODE

Many TENS units allow the clinician to use a "modulation" mode to decrease accommodation to the stimulation. This is most often used with sensory TENS because the large-diameter nerve fibers that are targeted with this type of stimulation accommodate quickly. Some manufacturers modulate the amplitude, the pulse rate, or the phase duration, usually by varying the parameter by 20% above and below the preset value. Different parameters may be modulated, depending on the device. Some TENS units allow modulation of amplitude, phase duration, or pulse rate, and some units are "multimodulated," which means two or more parameters are modulated (see figure 8.4).

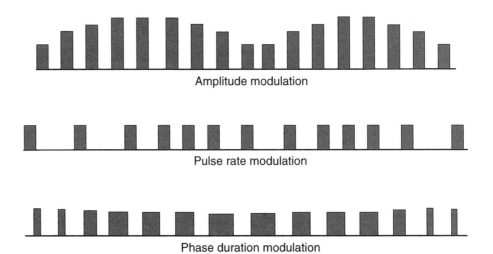

Amplitude modulation

Pulse rate modulation

Phase duration modulation

Figure 8.4 Modulation mode. Examples of modulation of the waveform include amplitude modulation, pulse rate modulation, and phase duration modulation. Modulation of the waveform helps to reduce accommodation.

Name_____   Date_____

Activities

1. Practice setting up different types of electrical stimulators with the various modes of TENS. Note that some machines have preset parameters that make them more suitable for a specific type of TENS. Set up a volunteer on sensory, motor, and noxious TENS.

2. Practice point location and stimulation with noxious TENS. Use the charts pictured in the Muscle Spasm Lab (lab 9) to help localize points.

3. Create a protocol for teaching an athlete or athletic trainer who is traveling with a team how to use the portable TENS unit, and write it below.

4. With the following patient types, demonstrate, discuss, and note in your manual (a) the electrode placement, (b) the mode of TENS treatment, and (c) the length of treatment.

   • Low back pain with radiating pain into the posterior thigh.

   • Acute shoulder dislocation.

   • Rehabilitating hamstring injury that continues to ache. The athlete has been able to return to practice.

   • Spasm in the upper trap and cervical region that limits the athlete's head movement.

   • Shin splints that prevent participation.

   • Patellar tendinitis.

LAB 9

Management of Muscle Spasm

Review material from chapter 6, pages 88 to 99, of the textbook before you complete this lab.

OBJECTIVES

- You will understand that there are numerous methods for treating muscle spasm, including ice or heat and manual therapies. This lab emphasizes the different uses of TENS to treat muscle spasm.

- You will understand that a complete musculoskeletal evaluation is essential to determine the pathology of the injury. Treatment of pain should be focused on resolving the problem rather than merely treating the symptoms.

- You will be introduced to the treatment of trigger and acupuncture points with electrical stimulation.

TREATMENT OF MUSCLE SPASM

There are numerous methods to treat muscle spasm with modalities. Heat and ice indirectly influence the muscle spindle, which is a sensory organ located in parallel with the skeletal muscle fibers. The muscle spindle is responsible for the stretch reflex, which causes the muscle to contract. Any factor that decreases sensitivity of the muscle spindle will decrease the resting tone of the muscle and promote relaxation of the muscle. If the muscle can be relaxed temporarily, the pathology can be addressed so that the pain–spasm cycle can be broken. For example, if there is a cervical facet sprain leading to increased tone in the shoulders and neck, modalities can modify the pain or spasm so that range-of-motion exercise or joint mobilization can be tolerated, which ultimately may rectify the problem.

There are several methods to decrease muscle spasm by using electrical stimulation. These examples are not exclusive. Any type of pain modulation technique using TENS can be used to reduce pain. The clinician should use experience and be ready to modify his or her technique to focus the treatment on the individual case. You should experiment with several methods to treat muscle spasm.

A complete musculoskeletal evaluation is essential to determine the pathology of the injury. Treatment of pain should be focused on resolving the problem rather than merely treating the symptoms. As the pain is reduced from the application of modalities, treatment should include therapeutic exercise to correct the problem.

TENS

TENS relieves pain and is effective in reducing the pain–spasm cycle. Once the pain is minimized with electrical stimulation, the athlete should be instructed in therapeutic exercise to resolve the condition. Sensory, motor, and noxious TENS treatments can be used depending on the situation. See lab 8 for parameters for each technique.

FATIGUE THE MUSCLE

If the muscle becomes fatigued, then theoretically it should relax after the treatment. The electrical stimulation is applied with a strong current (long phase duration and high, tolerable intensity). The stimulation is applied at a pulse rate at greater than tetany to create a strong contraction. The stimulation can last 10 to 30 min. Therapeutic exercise should follow the treatment to prevent the spasm from returning.

Fatigue

- Phase duration: > 250 μs
- Pulse rate: > 50 pps
- Amplitude: strong, comfortable contraction

- Type of current: any continuous
- Electrodes: over motor point of muscle

CONTRACT–RELAX

Another method of decreasing muscle spasm is to use the contract–relax technique for reciprocal inhibition. By creating a strong contraction with electrical stimulation, the Golgi tendon organ is excited. This inhibits the muscle being stimulated so that the muscle then relaxes. A duty cycle is imposed so that the contraction and relaxation are alternated: 15 sec on and 15 sec off is typical. This treatment may last 20 to 30 min while the amplitude of the current is increased gradually so that strong contractions are maintained. It is imperative that the amplitude be increased only during the "on" phase rather than during the rest cycle.

Contract–Relax:

- Phase duration: > 250 μs
- Pulse rate: > 50 pps
- Amplitude: strong, comfortable contraction
- Type of current: any
- Duty cycle: 1:1
- Electrodes: over motor point of muscle

ACUPUNTURE POINT STIMULATION

Eastern medicine theory uses the stimulation of acupuncture points to decrease pain. This method has been used with good empirical results for pain reduction, but few data substantiate its use. Figures 9.1 to 9.4 can be used to help locate commonly

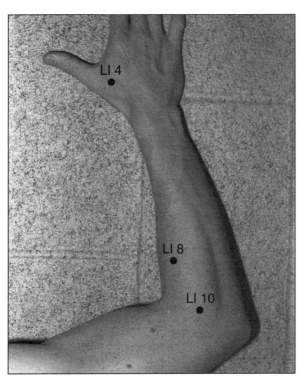
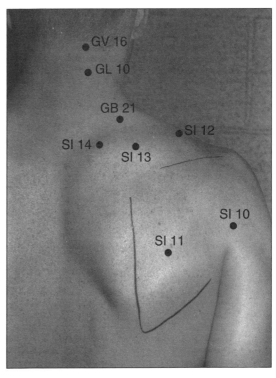

a

b

■ **Figure 9.1**   (a) Shoulder pain: LI 4—In the webspace of the first interosseous muscle near the radial aspect of the second metacarpal; LI 10—With the elbow flexed to 90°, two body inches below transverse cubital crease in the extensor mass. (b) Shoulder pain: SI 10—With the arm at the side, directly above the posterior axillary folder in the posterior joint capsule; SI 11—In the center of the infraspinatus muscle midway between the spine of the scapula and the inferior angle of the scapula; SI 13—At the superior, medial aspect of the scapula in the insertion of the levator scapula muscle; Cervical or thoracic pain: SI 12—In the center of the suprascapular fossa in the supraspinatus muscle; SI 14—Three body inches lateral to the spinous process of the first thoracic vertebra, but in line with the medial border of the scapula; GB 21—Midway between C 7 or T 1 disc space and the tip of the acromion at the highest point in the shoulder; GV 16—Directly below occipital protuberance in the midline; BL 10—Just lateral to the insertion of the trapezius muscle at the level of the transverse process between the first and second vertebrae.

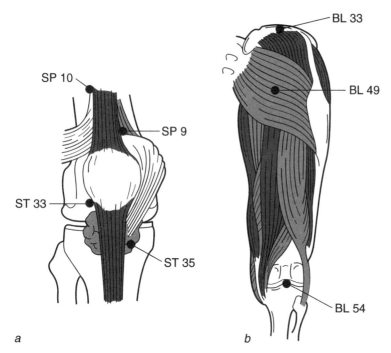

▌ Figure 9.2 *(a)* Knee pain: SP 9—In the depression on the lower aspect of the tibial flare, just lateral to the tibial tuberosity; SP 10—Two body inches above the superior border of the patella at the center of the vastus medialis muscle; ST 33—Three body inches above the superior lateral border of the patella; ST 35—With the knee flexed, find the depression lateral to the patellar tendon at the joint line; *(b)* Knee pain: BL 54—In the center of the popliteal fossa between the semitendinosus and biceps femoris tendons.

Adapted, by permission, from B. Behnke, 2001, *Kinetic anatomy* (Champaign, IL: Human Kinetics), 213.

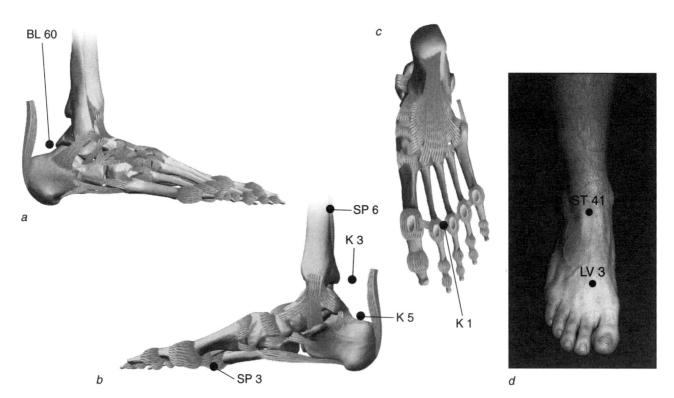

▌ Figure 9.3 *(a)* Ankle pain: BL 60—Midway between the inferior aspect of the lateral malleolus and the achilles tendon (just posterior to the talus); *(b)* ankle pain: SP 6—Three body inches above the tip of the medial malleolus on the posterior tibial border; K 3—Midway between the posterior aspect of the medial malleolus and the achilles tendon; K 5—Posterior to the flexor hallicus longus tendon in the depression between the achilles tendon and calcaneous; SP 3—On the medial aspect of the foot, posterior and inferior to the head of the first metacarpal; *(c)* ankle pain: K 1—Flex the toes at the transverse crease between the second and third metatarsophalangeal joints on the plantar aspect of the foot; *(d)* ankle pain: ST 41—Midpoint of the transmalleolar crease between the tendons of the extensor digitorum longus and extensor hallicus longus; LV 3—Proximal to the crease between the first and second toes at the interosseus muscle.

Parts a through c were adapted, by permission, from B. Behnke, 2001, *Kinetic anatomy* (Champaign, IL: Human Kinetics), 214.

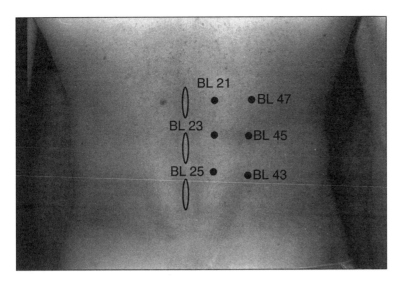

I Figure 9.4 Low back pain: bladder meridian—point parallel to spin (BL21-47) in two rows on each side two and four body inches from the spinous processes; BL 49—In the center of the gluteus max; BL 54—In the center of the popliteal fossa between the semitendinosus and biceps femoris tendons (BL 49 and BL 54 appear in figure 9.2b).

treated points. The points that are described for each joint can be stimulated depending on the specific problem. For example, when there is pain and spasm in the shoulder, stimulate all points listed for shoulder pathology. The cervical points may be included, depending on whether there is involvement in the neck. Points should be stimulated from distal to proximal, and if there is bilateral pain, stimulate all points on one side before progressing to the opposite side. Stimulation of auricular points in the ear also have been described in the literature as an effective means to decrease pain, but this is beyond the scope of this lab.

The explanation of point stimulation using noxious pain modulation is included in lab 8.

Name_____   Date_____

Activities

1. Set up a volunteer on the different methods to treat muscle spasm in the cervical, thoracic, or lumbar spine. Demonstrate the TENS methods and the fatigue, contract—relax, and acupuncture point stimulation techniques.

2. Locate some of the acupuncture points in figures 9.1 through 9.4—palpate the points and practice shiatsu acupressure. This is commonly used in massage to treat pain.

3. Note that the most important aspect of pain relief from muscle spasm is to find the cause of the pain. On a volunteer, evaluate posture and stress, which may contribute to upper thoracic and cervical trigger points. Address range of motion of muscles and joint mechanics that may contribute to the recurrence of pain. Note your findings here.

LAB 10

Neuromuscular Electrical Stimulation

Review material from chapter 8, pages 138 to 141 of the textbook, before you complete this lab.

OBJECTIVES

- You will understand when neuromuscular electrical stimulation (NMES) is indicated.

- You will understand the differences in an electrically produced contraction compared with a natural, physiological contraction.

- You will understand that duty cycle is a feature of an electrical stimulator that is critical for NMES application.

- You will understand what parameters affect the neuromuscular treatment.

- You will understand that for the muscle to be trained to perform an increased level of work, the force of the muscle must be high enough to elicit a force equal to 40 to 60% of the maximal voluntary force.

- You will understand that because the contraction cannot be inhibited, joints should be protected from hyperextension and joint jamming.

MUSCLE STRENGTHENING VERSUS FORCE-CAPACITY ENHANCEMENT

For a muscle to become stronger, a load must be placed on the muscle and adaptation must occur. Strength is measured by an increased ability to do work, usually by the ability to lift weights or produce more force. For strength to increase merely by using electrical stimulation, the stimulation must be as strong as imposing a similar overload as exercise. Currier (1991) reported that a force equal to 40 to 60% of the maximal voluntary force must be imposed with electrical stimulation for strengthening to occur. For example, if the athlete is able to lift 20 lb with the biceps volitionally, to strengthen the muscle electrically the stimulation should be strong enough to lift 8 to 12 lb. This level of electrical stimulation is rarely tolerable, and in normal situations, it is easier to exercise rather than use electrical stimulation for muscle strengthening.

In an injured population, electrical stimulation can assist neuromuscular function. If a muscle is inhibited from effusion or prolonged immobilization, electrical stimulation can be used to teach the athlete to contract the muscle. In this manner, the force capacity or ability of the muscle to contract is enhanced, but the muscle is not truly "strengthened." Electrical muscle stimulation always occurs through the motor nerve rather than by depolarizing the muscle membrane directly whenever the peripheral nerve is intact. Therefore, although muscle contraction is the goal, the technique is termed *neuromuscular electrical stimulation*, or NMES.

NMES can be used in sports medicine for muscle re-education following injury or surgery, to reduce disuse atrophy with immobilization, or to augment the function of an impaired muscle (functional electrical stimulation). For example, NMES may be used to assist dorsiflexion with foot-drop. Additionally, NMES may be used for focal stimulation of a weakness (e.g., stimulation of paraspinals on the convex side of scoliosis).

Table 10.1 lists differences between physiological and electrical muscle contractions.

Table 10.1   Differences Between Physiological and Electrical Muscle Contractions

	Physiological	Electrical
Order of recruitment	Slow-twitch fibers are excited first. Fast-twitch fibers are excited if increased force is required, preserving energy.	Larger-diameter, fast-twitch fibers are recruited first because they have a lower capacitance. Slow-twitch fibers are recruited if the stimulation is increased.
Synchrony of firing	There is asynchronous firing to promote a continuous contraction. This reduces the potential for fatigue of any one motor unit.	There is synchronous firing depending on the frequency of the stimulation. The contraction continues until the stimulation is off.
Inhibition	If the stimulation is strong, the Golgi tendon organ (GTO) will cause inhibition, which relaxes the muscle to prevent too strong of a contraction.	The GTO is excited, but inhibition of the alpha motor neuron is overcome because of direct stimulation of the peripheral nerve.
Fatigue	There is minimal fatigue because of the order of recruitment and asynchrony of firing of motor units.	The muscle fatigues rapidly from the fast-twitch fiber recruitment, which uses the phosphocreatine energy system, and from the synchronous nature of the firing.

FATIGUE AND NMES

Electrically produced contractions cause greater fatigue than physiological contractions, primarily because of the energy system used in the fast-twitch fibers. To reduce fatigue with electrical stimulation, a duty cycle or rest time must be imposed. Generally, a 1:5 on to off ratio is required to allow enough time to regenerate the local energy used for the contraction. The phosphocreatine energy system is depleted rapidly (in 10-15 sec) and requires 30 sec to 1 min to replace. The rest time allows quality contractions to be produced throughout the treatment. When NMES is used for muscle re-education or to promote quality muscle function, generally a 10-sec contraction is followed by a 45- to 50-sec rest time. As the athlete accommodates to the overload (after 1-2 weeks of training), the rest time can be reduced to 30 sec. Because of muscle fatigue, the duty cycle is probably the most important feature of a neuromuscular stimulator.

NMES PARAMETERS

The electrical stimulator's parameters of phase duration, pulse frequency, amplitude, and duty cycle can be adjusted to optimize the NMES treatment.

The phase duration with NMES should be high enough to overcome the capacitance of motor nerve fibers. Although the capacitance of these motor fibers is low, these fibers are deep and a high phase duration is recommended (250-300 μs) to increase recruitment of many motor units.

Because the goal is to produce a tetanous contraction, the pulse rate should be 35 to 50 pps. Usually 50 pps is used. Higher frequencies (more than 100 pps) do not cause a stronger contraction and promote early fatigue.

The amplitude with NMES depends on the goal of the treatment. If the purpose is to teach the athlete to contract the muscle, then the intensity should produce a strong, tolerable contraction. The athlete should superimpose a voluntary contraction with the electrical contraction whenever possible to enhance the force production. If the goal is strengthening the muscle, then the amplitude should be 40 to 60% of the maximal volitional force.

As described previously, the duty cycle is probably the most important parameter in NMES treatment because the electrically produced contractions cause more fatigue than exogenous contractions. The duty cycle should be 1:5 (10 sec on and 50 sec off) in the initial treatments, and as the athlete adapts to the stimulation, the duty cycle can be reduced to 1:3. The on time does not include the ramp time, so if a long ramp time is desired, increase the on time. For example, if the on time is 10 sec but there is a 3-sec ramp, then the maximal intensity is only on for 7 sec. Increase the on time in this case to 13 sec so that there is a maximal contraction for the full 10 sec.

TYPES OF NEUROMUSCULAR ELECTRICAL STIMULATORS

Any machine can be used as long as there is a duty cycle control. Ideally, the unit should be able to produce a strong, tetanous contraction. Commonly a *Russian stimulator* is used, which has unique parameters that were popularized by Kots, a Russian researcher who presented impressive results about muscle strengthening with electrical stimulation in 1977. The Russian stimulator parameters are preset and cannot be adjusted to vary the treatment.

**Russian Stimulator Parameters
(Time-Modulated, Medium-Frequency AC Stimulation)**

- Sinusoidal AC current with a carrier frequency of 2500 Hz
- Bursted or "time-modulated" with a 10 ms "on" time and 10 ms "off" time, which ultimately results in a 50 burst per minute frequency
- Duty cycle preset at 10 sec on and 50 sec off (with a 2- to 3-sec ramp)

NMES APPLICATION

The following is an example of a stimulation protocol for the quadriceps muscle. Explain the treatment protocol to the athlete, encouraging him or her to increase the current intensity for as strong a contraction as can be tolerated. Also encourage the athlete to superimpose a volitional contraction in conjunction with the stimulation.

Place one electrode over the femoral nerve in the femoral triangle and the other over the distal quadriceps proximal to the patella. Position the athlete in a device such as an orthotron, which adds isometric resistance to the contraction and limits the complete excursion of the limb. Avoid terminal extension to prevent joint "jamming" and soft tissue damage. The optimal knee angle to obtain maximal quadriceps muscle force by using NMES is 60° of knee flexion.

Treatment parameters may vary according to the type of unit used. The phase duration is often preset; otherwise, select 200 to 300 µs. The pulse frequency is also often preset, but if it is adjustable, select 40 to 50 Hz (30-40 Hz postoperatively) for tetany. Adjust the amplitude and increase it to tolerance of a maximal contraction. Make sure that the amplitude is adjusted only when the stimulation is "on" rather than during the rest phase. Set the duty cycle at 15 sec on and 50 sec off (this is preset on some units, otherwise use a 1:5 on/off ratio). Set the ramp time at 3 to 5 sec.

NMES Parameters

- Phase duration: often preset, otherwise 200 to 300 µs
- Frequency: often preset, otherwise 40 to 50 Hz (30-40 Hz postoperatively)
- Amplitude: adjusted and increased to tolerance of a maximal contraction
- Duty cycle: 15 sec on/50 sec off (a 1:5 on/off ratio)
- Ramp time: 3 to 5 sec

The treatment duration may vary according to the type of neuromuscular stimulator being used and the goal of the treatment. For example, the larger clinical models only require 10 to 15 contractions when maximally tolerated contractions are elicited. However, when you are "teaching" the athlete to contract a muscle after a surgical procedure, a greater number of submaximal contractions can be done. When using home portable units, the treatment can be repeated up to three times a day for up to 1 h, although overfatigue of the muscle groups should be discouraged. Generally these units do not elicit a maximal contraction (see figure 10.1).

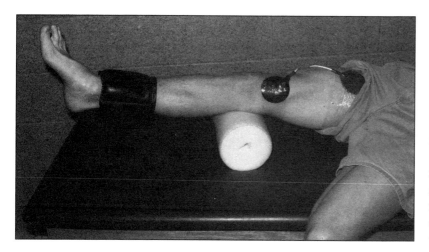

Figure 10.1 NMES for muscle re-education. Use the electrical stimulation to teach the athlete how to contract the muscle after an injury or surgery. Active exercise with the stimulation is encouraged.

Place the athlete in a position to allow the best contraction of the muscle. If there is a deficit in the muscle function in part of the range, such as with an extension lag of the knee, then the muscle should be strengthened in the weak aspect of the range (see figure 10.2).

If reciprocal stimulation of agonist/antagonist muscle groups is desired, position the joint so that both muscle groups can benefit. This is generally in the midrange of the joint motion.

When you are attempting to increase the force generated by the muscle with augmentation of electrical stimulation, the end range of the joint should be blocked. This position minimizes potential injury to the joint, because the inhibition caused normally by the Golgi tendon organ is unable to take place as long as the stimulation is on. Blocking terminal extension also prevents hyperextension of the joint.

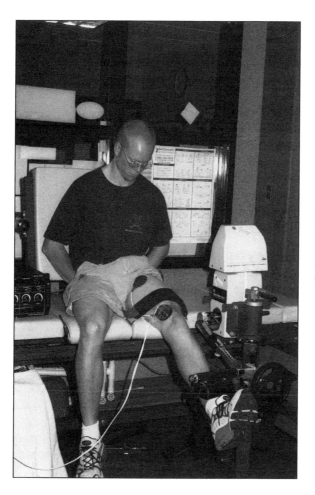

Figure 10.2 NMES for force-capacity enhancement. Block terminal extension to protect the joint. Use a concomitant maximal volitional contraction.

Name_____ Date_____

Activities

1. Examine the machines available and discuss and note below which are appropriate for NMES. Determine which machines have the optimal parameters.

2. Set up a volunteer on an isokinetic device so that the dynamometer can measure the force output. Have the person perform a maximal isometric contraction and measure the force. Apply the NMES on the quadriceps muscle, and increase the intensity to tolerance. Try to increase the intensity to 50% of the maximal isometric contraction. Note your findings here.

3. Using patient case studies, discuss when NMES should be used. Note the position, amplitude, phase duration, pulse rate, duty cycle, and length of treatment in the space provided.

   Case A: Three weeks after an anterior cruciate ligament reconstruction, the athlete continues to have a 15° extension lag. No pain is associated with the neuromuscular dysfunction.

   Case B: Five days after arthroscopic meniscectomy, an athlete has difficulty generating an effective quad set.

   Case C: During a shoulder rehabilitation, you notice that an athlete has difficulty stabilizing the scapula during arm elevation. There is weakness of the lower trap.

   Case D: An athlete has fractured her femur. She has a previous history of knee instability, and the physician has agreed to cut a "window" in the long-leg cast to allow NMES to minimize quad atrophy during immobilization.

4. Use NMES to promote elbow range of motion. Demonstrate the technique you would recommend, and note this here.

LAB 11

Interferential Current

Review material from chapter 8, pages 143 to 144 of the textbook, before you complete this lab.

OBJECTIVES

- You will understand the benefits of medium-frequency current.

- You will understand that medium-frequency currents require modulation to produce biologically active currents.

- You will understand Wedenski's inhibition.

- You will understand the difference between interferential currents and "premodulated" interferential currents.

INTERFERENTIAL STIMULATION

Interferential stimulation is another form of TENS used for pain relief, increased circulation, and muscle stimulation. Interferential current simultaneously applies two medium-frequency currents to achieve deeper penetration of the stimulation. Medium- and high-frequency currents reduce the skin impedance that minimizes the penetration of low-frequency currents. Medium-frequency currents must be modulated; otherwise, there is minimal or no response in the tissues. Typical modulation techniques include the incorporation of an internal duty cycle as with Russian stimulation or interfering the current to create a resultant "beat" frequency (see figure 11.1).

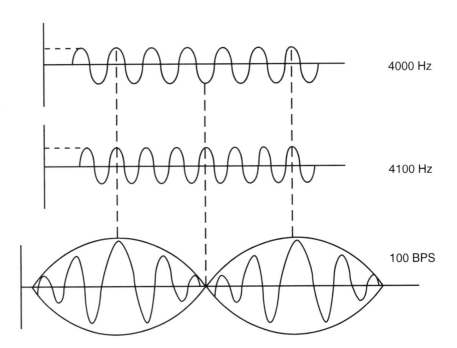

■ Figure 11.1   Interferential stimulation. Two different medium-frequency currents are superimposed so that there is augmentation and attenuation of the currents. The resultant frequency is the beat frequency and is the difference between the two carrier frequencies.

To modulate the medium frequency to a range that can create an action potential in the tissues, two slightly different medium-frequency (within the range of 1000-10000 Hz) sinusoidal wave currents are applied at the same time. Their waveforms are superimposed on each other, which causes interference. Interference creates points of augmentation and attenuates the phases where peaks and valleys are added together. The interference results in the modulation of a "beat" mode with a frequency that ranges from 1 to 100 beats per second (bps), which is well within the conventional low-frequency range. The beat frequency is determined by the difference between the two carrier frequencies. For example, carrier frequencies of 4000 and 4150 Hz will have a beat frequency of 150 bps, or frequencies of 2500 and 2550 Hz will have a beat frequency of 50 bps.

The medium-frequency currents used with interferential units can cause a cutaneous nerve inhibition, as with the action potential block mode of TENS. This action potential failure is known as Wedenski's inhibition and occurs as the stimulation is applied too fast for the refractory period of the nerve. At a frequency of 5000 Hz, the membrane is unable to stabilize, and the continuous function of the sodium–potassium pump causes an inhibitory effect. Wedenski's inhibition can be demonstrated by noting the anesthesia between the electrodes during medium-frequency stimulation. The patient should not be able to discriminate sharp or dull sensations between the electrodes during stimulation.

The frequency of the beats can vary by changing one of the two carrier frequencies. The beat frequency, not the carrier frequencies, affects the tissues, and changes in this parameter alter the stimulation responses. The number of muscle twitches is greater as the beat frequency increases, until a tetanic contraction is attained. Some units have a feature that constantly changes the frequency of one of the carrier currents while the other remains constant. This mode is a *sweep frequency*, which causes a rhythmic change throughout a range of frequencies. The purpose of the rhythmic mode is to reduce accommodation. Because the stimulation continuously changes, the body cannot adapt to it, and so the sweep frequency provides a more effective stimulation.

Some models include a rotating vector system that periodically changes the orientation of the electrical field 45° to further reduce accommodation. The efficacy of this modification has not been substantiated.

The beat frequency is selected according to the condition to be treated. A frequency of 60 to 100 bps is used for sensory TENS, 50 to 60 bps for muscle contraction, and 2 to 4 bps for motor TENS.

Four electrodes should be used for an interferential treatment, two for each carrier current. The electrodes of each current are placed diagonally over the treatment site. The area to be treated should be surrounded by the electrodes if it is an extremity or joint. If the treatment area is large, such as the low back, the electrodes should be placed all on one surface. Some interferential units also offer suction electrodes, in which a mild vacuum is created under the electrode to allow it to stick to the body part. These electrodes are convenient because they do not have to be strapped down, and they stay in place throughout the treatment.

The passage of current through the tissues does not occur linearly between the electrodes but creates an electrical field. This field is purported to be shaped in a cloverleaf pattern situated three-dimensionally between the electrodes. If the conductivity of the tissues was uniform, this perfectly formed electrical field would occur with the maximal current concentration in the central region between the electrodes. However, differences in tissue impedance affect the location of the electrical field and the degree of superposition of currents. Therefore, the concentration of current is not always centralized. To maximize the probability of properly placed electrodes and subsequent electrical fields, adjust the electrodes so that maximal intensity is perceived in the painful region (see figure 11.2).

Interferential stimulation can be used with other modalities. Ice or heat can be used in conjunction with the stimulation, although this is sometimes difficult with the suction electrodes. Treatment durations are dictated by the goal of treatment: pain relief, muscle re-education, muscle spasm reduction, and so forth. Interferential units have been shown to reduce pain and edema posttraumatically.

Contraindications to using interferential stimulators are the same for any other form of TENS, but caution should be taken when using interferential machines in

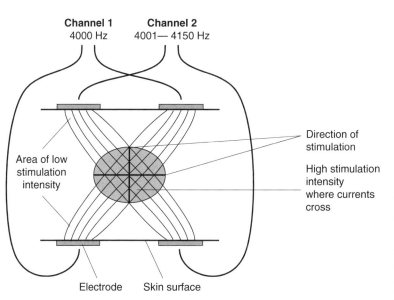

■ Figure 11.2 Stimulation produced with interferential current using four electrodes.

Reprinted, by permission, from Dynatronics Corporation, "Interferential and premodual: Interferential (quadpolar) therapy," *Dynation 950plus and 650plus* (Salt Lake City: author).

the proximity of diathermy units. The electrical field generated can cause power surges in the electrical modalities.

APPLICATION

Turn on the power to the interferential machine before setting up electrodes. This prevents a power surge from transmitting to the patient when powering on. Select the interferential mode if the unit has multiple options of stimulation parameters. There may be an option of selecting the carrier frequency. Generally your decision will be determined by your treatment goal. For example, if there are options of 2500 Hz and 5000 Hz, remember that the higher the frequency, generally the better the depth of penetration (according to the formula that affects impedance). However, a 2500-Hz current has a phase duration of 200 μs (1/2500 = 400 μs; since the waveform is biphasic, each phase is 200 μs). A current with 5000 Hz has only a 100-μs phase duration. Therefore, if a longer phase duration is desired, which may be the case when using neuromuscular stimulation, select the lower carrier frequency.

Select the treatment frequency. This also will be dictated by the treatment goal. Use the appropriate treatment frequencies for the pain modulation theories, or set the frequency at tetany for neuromuscular stimulation. You may be able to select a frequency scan that modulates the frequency throughout a preset range to decrease accommodation. The treatment frequency is actually the difference in the two medium-frequency currents (e.g., 5000 Hz and 5100 Hz results in 100 bps).

Determine the duty cycle for the treatment. If the treatment is for pain, generally a continuous (no duty cycle) treatment is chosen. Neuromuscular treatments require a rest time, and both the on time and the off time should be selected as appropriate for the treatment.

Set up the electrodes. Moist sponges can be used to improve conductance. Two complete channels must be connected to the athlete. Ideally, the stimulation should cross between the electrodes. Firmly secure the electrodes to the athlete.

Begin to increase the intensity of the stimulation, one circuit at a time. When the intensity of the second circuit is increased, the perception of stimulation may change. Increase each circuit a little at a time while getting feedback from the athlete about the location of maximal stimulation and the comfort level of the current. Adjust amplitude only when the duty cycle is on, rather than during the rest phase.

Some interferential units allow the clinician to "move" the current to allow better placement of the stimulation. This may be done with a joystick or a finger panel, and it requires feedback from the athlete, which is called a vector scan. Vector scan can be selected if the treatment site cannot be isolated. One circuit will intrinsically vary its amplitude, changing the location of maximal stimulation. This will reduce the time the treatment current is at the injury site, so a longer treatment duration is recommended. Check the athlete for comfort during the treatment, and make adjustments as necessary.

PREMODULATED INTERFERENTIAL STIMULATION

Premodulated interferential stimulation is designed to make interferential stimulation easier to set up. The premise is that the two medium-frequency currents are crossed inside the machine so that only two electrodes, or one channel, is necessary for the treatment. However, the benefit of interferential stimulation is that by applying two medium-frequency currents to the skin, the beat frequency will be produced inside the body at the location of the pathology. By crossing the currents before applying them to the body, the treatment becomes very similar to time-modulated AC or burst mode TENS (see lab 6). The medium frequency is modified to a biologically active low frequency before it reaches the body. This method is a very effective method of TENS, because both sensory and motor pain modulation stimulation can be done.

APPLICATION OF PREMODULATED INTERFERENTIAL

Determine your treatment goal, for example, sensory pain modulation, muscle spasm reduction by fatigue, or neuromuscular stimulation. Select premodulation (sometimes abbreviated "Pre-Mod" on the unit). Adjust the treatment frequency and duty cycle depending on the treatment goal.

Attach one channel (two electrodes) securely to the athlete, and increase the intensity to the desired level depending on the treatment goal.

Name_____   Date_____

Activities

1. In small groups, discuss interferential current and time-modulated AC currents (discussed in lab 6). Draw the waveforms used with medium-frequency therapy. Discuss and note below why medium-frequency currents require modulation.

2. Using a quadripolar electrode configuration for interferential current, experiment with electrode positioning. Fill a bucket with water, and tape electrodes on opposite sides of the bucket. Turn up the stimulation on both channels and, with a volunteer's finger, find the area of highest stimulation in the water. Note that the three-dimensional area of stimulation is centrally concentrated in the uniform bucket of water, but discuss and note below how that might change in heterogeneous tissues of the body.

3. Set up a volunteer with interferential and use a vector-scan technique to change the location of the maximal stimulation. Using a paper clip, test the sensation between the electrodes and note your results here.

4. Practice using interferential and premodulated interferential stimulation and note your results here.

LAB 12

High-Voltage Stimulation

Review material from chapter 8, pages 142 to 143 of the textbook, before you complete this lab.

OBJECTIVES

- You will understand the specific type of waveform used in high-voltage stimulation.

- You will understand the benefits of using high voltage when other electrical stimulators are available.

- You will understand the implications of polarity and electrical-field production with a monophasic current.

High-voltage stimulators have two distinct specifications: they must be able to transmit a voltage in excess of 100 V, and they must use a twin peak, monophasic waveform. The 100 V delineation is an arbitrarily set value that demarcates high- and low-voltage units. The major claim for this type of unit is that the high voltage allows deeper penetration of the energy and that the short phase duration of the twin peaks does not allow the capacitance of smaller sensory fibers (A-delta or C fibers) to be stimulated, resulting in greater comfort (see figure 12.1).

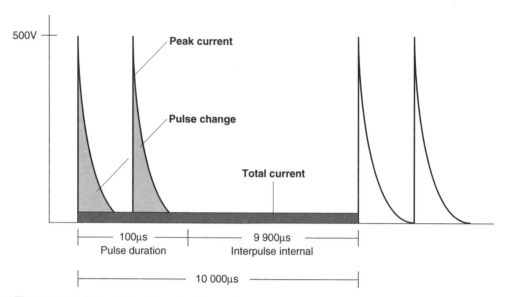

■ Figure 12.1 Twin peak, monophasic waveform.
Reprinted, by permission, from C.R. Denegar, 2000, *Therapeutic modalities for athletic injuries* (Champaign, IL: Human Kinetics), 142.

Because the stimulator is monophasic, there is a polarity difference in the electrodes, allowing the clinician to choose a positive or negative electrode for the treatment area. However, because the phase duration is so short, there are minimal physiochemical changes under the electrodes. High-voltage units are used clinically for pain control, edema reduction, tissue healing, and muscle spasm reduction. Muscle re-education can be done with high-voltage units if the stimulator allows a rest cycle.

The voltage amplitude available with most high-voltage machines ranges from 0 to 500 V. The amplitude, as with most electrical stimulators, is determined by patient comfort and the objective of the treatment (sensory or motor response). One feature of the high-voltage machine is that although the voltage is high, there is a low average current. It is, therefore, a very safe modality. The twin peak waveform allows the high peak but low average current. The pulse begins to decay almost immediately, and the second pulse begins before the first peak reaches the isoelectric line. The duration of both peaks together varies with each manufacturer but is generally between 50 and 120 μs. The phase duration is not adjustable by the clinician, which ensures the safety of the unit.

Many claims have been made about the relevance of the polarity control of high-voltage units, although the low average current minimizes any ion flux or physiochemical response. However, during healing, the wound emits a charge potential depending on the stage of healing. This potential is believed to be reinforced by applying the polarity of a like charge, either positive or negative, from the stimulator. This process promotes a stronger physiological response, which may enhance healing and edema reduction. However, the electrophoretic effect with this type of unit is negligible, especially with short treatment durations. The net ion flux across the membrane is minimal and self-limiting. The short phase durations cause only a minor shift in ion migration, and with the interpulse interval, the membrane can neutralize any change in the normal ion status. Iontophoresis cannot be performed with this unit because no net ion flux occurs. Several studies have addressed the possibility of edema reduction with high voltage, with inconclusive results.

The frequency range offered by most high-voltage units is from 2 to 120 pps. The frequency adjustment allows the incorporation of either sensory or motor TENS principles when pain tolerance is the goal. The variation in frequencies also allows the clinician to optimize parameters for either muscle pumping or muscle re-education.

Electrode placement for high voltage often uses the monopolar technique, although the bipolar can be used as well. The monopolar procedure uses one or more active electrodes and a larger dispersive electrode. The active electrodes are smaller in size and concentrate the current and, therefore, the level of stimulation. As the name implies, the dispersive electrode spreads the same amount of current over a larger surface area, causing minimal, if any, sensory perception under the dispersive electrode. The active electrodes are placed over the treatment site, and the dispersive electrode is placed on a site distant to the treatment area. Because the distance between electrodes is increased with the monopolar method, there is potentially a deeper penetration of the current.

The bipolar technique, which uses equal-sized electrodes over the same treatment area, can also be used with high voltage. The larger electrode is replaced by a smaller one, although the cord must be plugged into the dispersive socket in the unit; otherwise, the circuit is not complete (see figure 12.2).

A key feature of the high-voltage unit is its ability to be used with appendage-submersion treatments. Submersion is a preferred method of treatment for acute ankle injuries because it provides circumferential cooling and sensory TENS for irregular surfaces. Even though the extremity is in a dependent position, the submersion method allows active range of motion during the treatment. The active electrodes are placed in the cold water bath (55-65° F), and a 20- to 30-min treatment is applied. The treatment is followed by other modalities and exercise, as indicated for the condition. The treatment can be repeated several times throughout the day.

High-voltage stimulation with monophasic current has the same applications as other TENS units: sensory and motor pain modulation, improved blood flow, and edema reduction. High-voltage stimulation has the same contraindications as all

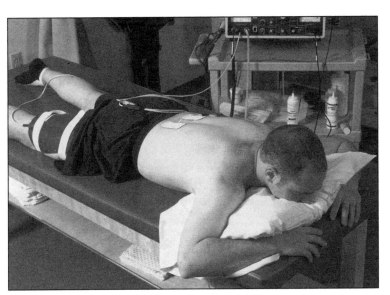

a

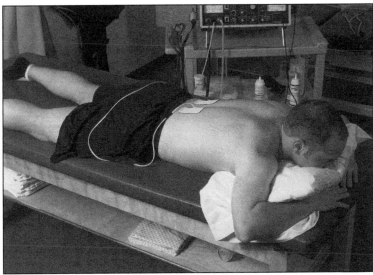

b

■ **Figure 12.2**
(a) Setups using a dispersive pad (monopolar) and *(b)* a small electrode (bipolar).

TENS methods and should not be used through the chest, whenever there is a cardiac pacemaker, or during pregnancy. High-voltage stimulation should not be used over the carotid sinus in the neck because of the proximity of the baroreceptors.

APPLICATION OF HIGH-VOLTAGE STIMULATION

The evaluation should delineate the goal of high-voltage stimulation. The high-voltage unit does not have an adjustable phase duration; therefore, strong contraction as with motor TENS may not be possible. See if your high-voltage stimulator has an adjustable duty cycle. If not, then the high-voltage stimulator cannot be used for NMES because there is no way to impose a rest time. The pulse frequency should be set depending on the goal of the treatment (sensory or motor TENS, muscle pumping, or muscle contraction). If the high-voltage stimulator is to be used in a water bath, ensure that ground fault circuit interrupters are in good working order.

From the evaluation, determine whether a monopolar or bipolar electrode configuration is desired. Set up the electrodes using the applicable technique. Make sure the dispersive pad is not causing transthoracic current.

Increase the amplitude to get the desired response (depending on the treatment goal—sensory or motor response). The high-voltage stimulator has a short phase duration, and the sensory nerves accommodate quickly to this stimulus. The amplitude may have to be increased periodically during the treatment. When the treatment time has ended, turn the amplitude back to zero and disconnect the electrodes. Evaluate the treatment response and inspect the skin. Return all electrodes, and power down the stimulator.

Name_____ Date_____

Activities

1. Discuss and note the waveform and characteristics that are unique to high-voltage stimulation. Compare this monophasic stimulator with a galvanic generator.

2. Demonstrate, discuss, and note methods with which high voltage can be used for pain relief and wound healing. Attempt to use high-voltage stimulation for the following:

   ☐ Sensory TENS

   ☐ Motor TENS

   ☐ NMES

   ☐ Muscle pumping for edema control

   ☐ Creating an electrical field for wound healing

3. Demonstrate the setup with either a monopolar or bipolar electrode configuration with high-voltage stimulation. With the following patient problems, note whether monopolar or bipolar would be advantageous.

   • Underwater stimulation for an acute ankle sprain

   • Patellar tendinitis

   • Deep thigh contusion

   • Pitting edema in the foot

   • Stimulation of a trigger point in the upper trap

   • Low back pain

LAB 13

Uses of Direct Current

Review material from chapter 8, pages 146 to 150 of the textbook, before you complete this lab.

OBJECTIVES

- You will be able to describe direct current stimulation and identify which machines produce this type of current.

- You will be able to describe the unique features of direct stimulation, specifically the polarity effects under each electrode.

- You will be able to apply iontophoresis.

- You will understand the principles of denervation and be able to apply direct current to denervated muscle.

DIRECT CURRENT STIMULATION

A direct current (DC) stimulator provides a continuous, unidirectional or monophasic current flow in a single direction for longer than 1 sec. Only a DC or galvanic stimulator has this unique waveform. There is no control of the phase duration or frequency on this machine, because these are not necessary. The maximal amplitude allowed often is limited, because DC has a high average current and can be dangerous.

Because DC is a monophasic current, there are polarity effects between the two electrodes. One electrode is always positive (the anode) and one electrode is always negative (cathode) (see table 13.1 for a comparison of positive and negative electrodes). When the direct current is applied, certain chemical effects occur that are dependent on the polarity of the electrode. These are the physiochemical effects of electrical stimulation and are a function of the high average current with DC stimulation.

Table 13.1   Polarity Effects With Galvanic Stimulation

Positive	Negative
Attracts acids	Attracts alkali
Repels alkali	Repels acids
Hardens tissue	Softens tissue
Contracts tissue	Dilates tissue
Stops hemorrhage	Increases hemorrhage
Diminishes congestion	Increases congestion
Sedating	Stimulating
Relieves pain in acute conditions by reducing congestion	Reduces pain in chronic conditions because of softening effect
Scars formed are hard and firm	Scars are soft and pliable

UNDERSTANDING IONTOPHORESIS

Iontophoresis is the process by which ions in solution are transferred through the intact skin via an electrical potential. Iontophoresis is based on the electrical principle that like charges are repelled. Therefore, the ions in solution (of similar charge) migrate away from the electrical source into the body. Iontophoresis is a noninvasive method to introduce drugs locally. Examples of some of the medications used in iontophoresis are listed in table 13.2. A DC generator is required for iontophoresis. Other monophasic stimulators have short phase durations, and the current does not flow long enough to cause physiochemical changes or a driving effect (see figure 13.1).

Commercially produced units for iontophoresis such as the Phoresor or Iontophor make the application of iontophoresis very easy. The following describes the procedure for using a commercial unit. Following the instructions of the specific model, explain the procedure to the athlete. Clean the treatment surface with either alcohol or soap and water. Fill the active electrode with the medication, and place it over the treatment site. Apply the dispersive pad, usually proximally.

Some units have a feature to alter the duration of the treatment depending on the intensity of current used. The clinician sets the milliamp-minutes on this type of

Table 13.2 Pathology and Recommended Ions Used With Iontophoresis

Condition	Medication	Polarity
Pain and inflammation	Salicylate	−
	Hydrocortisone	+
	Lidocane	+
	Dexamethasone	−
Calcium deposits	Acetic acid	−
Fungi	Copper	+
Adhesions	Chlorine	−
Edema	Magnesium sulfate	+
Spasms	Magnesium sulfate	+

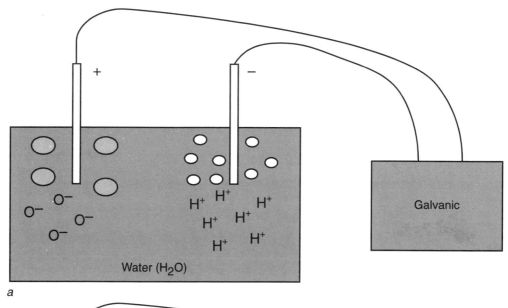

a

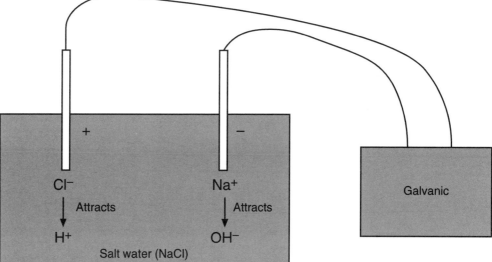

b

■ Figure 13.1 *(a)* Place each level of a galvanic stimulator into a container of water. Turn on the current and note the development of many small bubbles at the *negative* electrode (hydrogen ions) and the development of a few larger bubbles at the *positive* electrode (oxygen ions). *(b)* Place each lead into a container of salt water. The salt water dissociates in water into Na^+ and CL^- ions. The CL^- is attracted to the positive electrode, which forms HCL acid. The Na^+ is attracted to the negative electrode, which forms NaOH, a strong base. This is similar to what happens in the body.

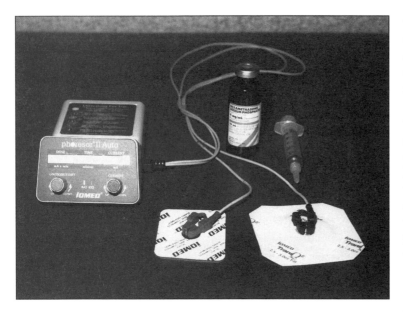

Figure 13.2 Commercial iontophoresis unit: small galvanic generator with one electrode that can be injected with the desired medication. The other electrode is dispersive.

unit. Increase the current 1 mA · min up to 4 to 5 mA, but always use patient comfort as a guideline. Inspect the skin and discard the electrodes after the treatment (see figures 13.2 and 13.3).

Iontophoresis can be done with a conventional low-voltage direct current stimulator, although the technique is not as easy. Explain the treatment to the athlete and ensure that the skin is clean and the integrity is good (i.e., no open wounds or abrasions). Prepare the electrodes or treatment baths. The pads should be well moistened (saturated but not dripping) with either tap water or medicinal solution. If you use an ointment, apply it underneath the electrode. Saturate a double layer of gauze with tap water or medicinal solution and place it over the treatment site. Place several layers of aluminum foil to make an electrode over the gauze, and connect the leads to the electrodes using alligator clips. Make sure no metal is touching the athlete.

Check the drug polarity, and use the electrode of like charge as the active electrode. Set the stimulator on continuous DC. The solution strength of the medication should be 1 to 5%, because higher concentrations are less effective and can seriously damage the skin. Make sure the solution is in the appropriate concentration before use.

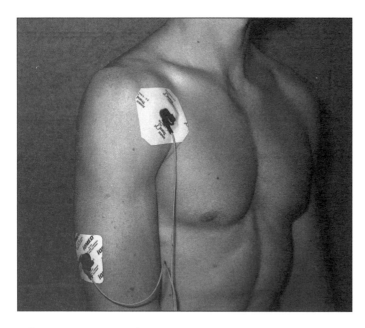

Figure 13.3 Iontophoresis treatment. The active electrode on the anterior aspect of the shoulder contains the medication.

Make the athlete comfortable and explain that he or she may experience a sensation of pins and needles that evolves into warmth. No discomfort or burning sensation should occur! Dosage is determined by the current intensity and duration. Once the paresthesia is perceived, increase the intensity 1 mA · min up to 5 mA. Skin resistance may decrease after several minutes of treatment, so the intensity may have to be decreased. The typical treatment duration is 15 to 20 min. If the intensity has to be reduced, use a longer treatment. When terminating the treatment, slowly reduce the intensity. Rinse the remaining solution and inspect the skin.

DENERVATED MUSCLE STIMULATION

Stimulation of denervated muscles is controversial since researchers have not been able to show an acceleration of nerve regrowth when stimulation is used. The goal of stimulation of denervated muscles, however, is not to attempt to accelerate the regrowth of the nerve, only to maintain the contractile function of the muscle while the nerve is regrowing. Electrically imposed contractions attempt to maintain the physiology and histology of the tissue and help to prevent some of the connective-tissue changes.

Denervated muscles require galvanic stimulation since the capacitance of the muscle is much higher than that of a nerve. Partially innervated muscles may be stimulated by a current with a shorter phase duration. A point stimulator should be used over the motor point, which is generally located in the muscle belly. Expect a twitch response since the muscle will be unable to hold the contraction. Only one action potential is possible per pulse. The muscle can be stimulated 5 to 10 times, 3 times per week. It is important not to fatigue the muscle, and stimulation should stop before the muscle is unable to be stimulated.

Many times the sensory loss from denervation does not correlate to the location of the denervated muscle. Therefore, the sensory nerves will be stimulated by the galvanic current. This stimulation may sting, but it should be tolerable. Gradually increase the stimulation at each point.

Name_____ Date_____

Discussion Questions

1. Using the following situations, discuss and note below whether denervated stimulation is appropriate in athletic training:

   Case A: An athlete punched his hand through a glass window and lacerated the motor branch of the median nerve in the thenar eminence. Motor points for the opponens and flexor pollicus brevis muscles should be stimulated.

   Case B: In a case of Bell's palsy, motor points of all muscles of facial expression should be stimulated five to eight times each.

   Case C: Ice was used indiscriminately at the lateral aspect of the knee, injuring the fibularis nerve and drop foot. Motor points for the anterior tibialis and extensor digitorum longus should be stimulated.

Activities

1. Place both leads of a DC generator into a glass of water. Turn the stimulator up to 1 mA and progressively increase to 5 mA. After about 15 min, examine the leads and the bubbles in the water. Which lead is suspected to be positive, and which is negative? Note your findings here.

2. Insert each lead of a galvanic stimulator into a hard-boiled egg. Turn up the intensity to 5 mA for 10 min. Note below what happens to the egg white at each lead.

3. With a DC stimulation, place a negative (black) electrode on the gastrocnemius and a positive (red) electrode on the thigh. Set up the unit on galvanic or DC stimulation. Allow current to flow for about 5 min, gradually increasing intensity

to 5 mA. Note responses and check the skin under the electrodes following treatment. Experiment with electrode sizes. How does this stimulation feel compared with biphasic TENS? Does the stimulation feel equal under each electrode? Note your findings here.

4. Iontophoresis

   a. Prepare a solution of salicylate (make sure the volunteer does not have an aspirin allergy).

   b. Soak gauze pads in the solution so that they are saturated but not dripping. Wrap the gauze around a metal electrode so that no metal is exposed to the skin. Attach to the unit via the negative pole with an alligator clip. The positive electrode is used as a dispersive and should be larger and placed proximal to the site.

   c. Turn up the intensity gradually to 5 mA. Note that the athlete should feel strong tingling, but the amplitude should be decreased if burning is perceived.

LAB 14

Ultrasound

Review material from chapter 9, pages 156 to 173 of the textbook, before you complete this lab.

OBJECTIVES

- You will be able to describe thermal and nonthermal uses of ultrasound.

- You will be able to examine an ultrasound machine to determine its frequency, effective radiating area, and beam nonuniformity ratio.

- You will understand the relationship between the sound head movement and the beam nonuniformity ratio.

- You will understand contraindications and precautions to the use of ultrasound.

- You will understand the dosage of ultrasound and how the frequency, intensity, duration, treatment area, and duty cycle affect the dosage.

- You will explore methods to improve consistency of ultrasound treatments.

Ultrasound is the application of high-frequency sound waves beyond human audibility. Although ultrasound is used diagnostically for various medical purposes, it has become an important therapeutic modality in physical medicine. The therapeutic application of ultrasound on soft tissues began in the United States in the 1950s and is now purportedly the most effective deep-heating modality used in physical therapy.

Ultrasound is very effective in providing heat to soft tissues because it operates with a minimal increase in superficial temperature. The mechanical energy causes ultrasound to also have nonthermal effects. The clinical uses of ultrasound are numerous in sports medicine. Thermal effects can increase tissue extensibility, which can increase range of motion when combined with a stretch or can be used to treat muscle spasm. Nonthermal effects include pain relief and reduction of inflammation, and ultrasound also may affect collagen production and alignment.

ULTRASOUND EQUIPMENT

The components of an ultrasound unit consist of an electrical generator, an oscillating circuit with a duty cycle selector, a coaxial cable, and the sound head, or transducer. The transducer contains the crystal that converts electrical energy to mechanical acoustical energy. The unit contains a timer that regulates the duration of the treatment and a power meter to provide information about the total watts (power) and the watts per square centimeter (intensity) that the unit is generating.

Ultrasound is produced by the conversion of electrical energy to acoustical energy by the reverse piezoelectric effect. The piezoelectric effect is the production of an electrical charge with deformation of a crystal. A reverse piezoelectric effect is the opposite—mechanically deforming a crystal by introducing an electrical current. The compression and expansion of the crystal result in a vibrational activity that ultimately creates the ultrasound. Each crystal has an inherent resonating frequency depending on its composition, diameter, and width. This resonating frequency occurs when the crystal's deformation and subsequent vibration are at a maximum for a given amount and rate of energy applied. Some crystals are capable of resonating at frequencies of both 1 and 3 MHz, eliminating the need to change transducers when changing frequencies. These units are more expensive but are more convenient and practical.

EFFECTIVE RADIATING AREA AND BEAM NONUNIFORMITY RATIO

Two factors that must be considered when referencing the transducer are the effective radiating area (ERA) and the beam nonuniformity ratio (BNR). These address the output characteristics of the crystals and can affect treatment parameters.

The ERA describes the surface area of the crystal that emits significant mechanical energy; the ERA is always smaller than the actual size of the crystal. The ERA is calculated by scanning the sound head 5 mm away from the radiating surface and measuring the areas that emit at least 5% of the maximal power output anywhere over the surface of the transducer. Any area that produces this minimal amount of energy is considered in the ERA. Transducers whose ERAs are close to the actual size of the transducer are generally better quality crystals and provide a more consistent treatment.

The clinician should be aware of the ERA when determining the dosage of ultrasound treatment. Intensity is determined by taking the total watts delivered divided by the ERA and is measured in watts per square centimeters.

$$\text{Intensity} = \frac{\text{watts (W)}}{\text{ERA (cm}^2)}$$

The ERA also determines the size of the area that can be treated effectively. When large surface areas are treated, the energy is dispersed over a broad area, which decreases the response. It is generally suggested to treat each area that is no larger than two to three times the size of the transducer for 5 min. Larger areas can be divided into treatment "fields" and each one treated for the appropriate duration. This method does not provide an effective thermal treatment for larger areas such as the paraspinal because one subfield may cool before exercise is initiated. Diathermy may be the modality of choice for providing deep heat to larger surface areas.

BNR is another measure of the consistency and quality of the crystal. Ultrasound energy is not consistent as it is emitted from the sound head. The meter displays the average intensity delivered (W/cm^2), but there may be regions that deliver much higher intensities in the beam. The BNR is the ratio of the highest intensity found in the ultrasound beam compared with the average intensity indicated on the power meter. A BNR of 6:1 indicates that intensities of 6.0 W/cm^2 can be found in the near-field region when the intensity is set at 1.0 W/cm^2. The lower the BNR, the better, although a BNR of 6:1 generally is considered acceptable. The higher the BNR, the greater the chance for "hot-spots" to be encountered, and the sound head must be kept moving at a faster pace to prevent the high-intensity location from being concentrated on one area.

NONTHERMAL EFFECTS

Therapeutic ultrasound has both nonthermal and thermal effects. The proposed nonthermal effects are increased membrane permeability and mechanical agitation. Acoustical streaming is the movement of fluids along boundaries of cell membrane that allows for increased ionic exchange through mechanical pressure of wave pulsing. Acoustical streaming has been proposed to increase fibroblastic activity. The effects of nonthermal ultrasound also are attributed to the propagation of vibration, which causes a micromassage. Stable cavitation and condensation and rarefaction of the cells occur, causing gas bubbles to expand and contract as the sound wave passes. The cavitation results in mechanical stimulation.

THERMAL EFFECTS

Thermal effects of ultrasound are attributed to the heat created by the mechanical agitation of the molecules. There are several theories concerning the benefits of thermal ultrasound. There may be increased blood flow with thermal ultrasound, although blood flow in muscles is under metabolic control rather than thermal influences. When soft tissue is heated, collagen extensibility increases due to decreased viscosity of ground substance in connective tissue. The thermal effects may increase the pain threshold of free nerve endings and increase the metabolism and enzymatic activity of cells.

It is important to understand the application of ultrasound and know what pathologies should not be treated with ultrasound. Ultrasound should not be used over any area of ischemia or inadequate blood flow, because the heat will not be dissipated. Continuous ultrasound should not be used on an area of inflammation because the increased heat exacerbates bleeding. Ultrasound should not be used over the eyes because of the possibility of cavitation of the vitreous humor. No modality, especially ultrasound, should be used over the pregnant uterus. Like superficial heat, ultrasound should not be used in the presence of cancer because it may exacerbate metastasis due to increased metabolism and the mechanical energy. Ultrasound should not be applied to the spinal cord after a laminectomy because of the possibility of cavitation in the central nervous system. Caution also should be used when treating areas with open epiphyses. Some studies have demonstrated premature closing of growth plates with high-intensity therapeutic ultrasound.

USING THE ULTRASOUND MACHINE

When using the ultrasound machine, athletic trainers need to understand the dosage of the ultrasound and how the frequency, intensity, duty cycle, and duration and size of treatment area affect the dosage. All of these parameters should be documented with each treatment.

FREQUENCY

Therapeutic ultrasound operates at the frequencies of approximately 1 MHz (mega = million) or up to 3 MHz. State-of-the-art synthetic crystals can be manufactured to provide almost any resonating frequency, but either 1 or 3 MHz is used most often in physical medicine. Having two available frequencies gives the clinician the option of choosing the frequency that is best suited for the tissue to be treated.

There is an inverse relationship between the frequency of ultrasound and the depth of penetration into the soft tissue. A 1-MHz ultrasound will dissipate 50% of its energy at a depth of 5 cm into soft tissue, whereas a 3-MHz unit will dissipate 50% of its energy at 1 cm depth. There are some variations in the depth of penetration with either frequency because tissues are not homogeneous. Tissues with a high protein content like muscle and nerve, for example, absorb more ultrasound energy, causing less penetration. The depth of penetration is determined by frequency, not by intensity of the ultrasound. Generally, superficial tissues such as the hand or patellar tendon are treated with 3-MHz ultrasound, and deeper structures such as the quadriceps muscle are treated with 1 MHz. Because ultrasound cannot penetrate through bone, there is less of a chance of periosteal irritation with 3-Mz ultrasound. A general rule is that if the target tissue is more than 1 inch deep, the 1-MHz frequency should be used. If the target tissue is more superficial than 1 inch, 3 MHz should be used.

INTENSITY

Intensity depends on the desired effects. For thermal effects, continuous wave ultrasound is used and intensities are generally higher. If nonthermal effects are desired, use pulsed ultrasound (20% and 50% duty cycles are available with most units) with lower intensities. Total output always depends on the athlete's tolerance and the amount of soft tissue coverage. Most units cannot exceed 3.0 W/cm².

For thermal effects, intensities should range from 1.0 to 2.0 W/cm². The intensity of ultrasound diminishes as it penetrates (termed *half-value thickness*). When determining the intensity, consider that dosage will have decreased by the time the energy reaches deeper target tissues.

For nonthermal effects, use the pulsed mode at similar intensities (remember there is a duty cycle, so the total energy will be much less). Use lower intensities with subacute injuries and higher with more chronic injuries.

Because higher frequencies (3 MHz) concentrate the energy in the superficial tissues, lower intensities generally are used. A general rule is to decrease the intensity by 0.3 to 0.5 W/cm² when using a higher frequency.

The half-value thickness is the depth of penetration in which one half of the intensity has been absorbed. Although the penetration of ultrasound depends on the frequency, consider the depth of the target tissue when determining the intensity. If the pathology is deep, choose the lower frequency and increase the intensity to make sure an adequate energy level reaches the target tissue. For example, for a thermal effect on a deep hamstring strain, 1 MHz ultrasound should be used. Because half of the energy attenuates in 3 cm, use the higher range of intensity (1.2-1.5 W/cm²).

Determining the intensity of ultrasound is difficult and takes practice. It is better to err with too little rather than too much energy. Most athletes are exercising, which adds heat and energy to the injured structure. Therefore, some athletic trainers choose to use lower dosages of ultrasound to minimize the deleterious effects of overstimulation.

DUTY CYCLE

Duty cycle depends on the goal of the treatment, either thermal or nonthermal. Basically, the energy is "turned off" periodically when pulsed ultrasound is used. The duty cycle is generally calculated as a percentage of the "on" time for ultrasound. For example, the duty cycle is the "on" time divided by the total time ("on" time plus the "off" time). Typically, 20% or 50% is used.

Duty cycle calculation (ultrasound)

$$\frac{\text{"on" time}}{\text{"on" + "off" time}} \quad \text{or} \quad \frac{2 \text{ ms}}{2 \text{ ms} + 8 \text{ ms}} = 20\%$$

Ultrasound duty cycles can be as low as 10% and as high as 100%, or continuous ultrasound. Pulsed ultrasound minimizes the both the thermal and nonthermal effects by decreasing the total energy output.

DURATION

The duration of the ultrasound treatment depends on the size of the treatment area. Do not try to cover an area larger than two to three times the size of the sound head (ERA) in a 5-min duration. Adjust the time for the size of the treatment area and the size of the sound head. When treating larger areas, divide the treatment area into fields of the appropriate size and treat each field individually. Exceptionally large areas such as the paraspinals of the back might require a type of therapy other than ultrasound (see figure 14.1).

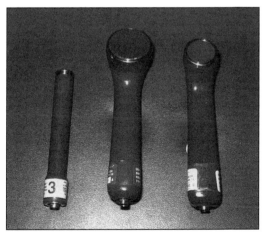 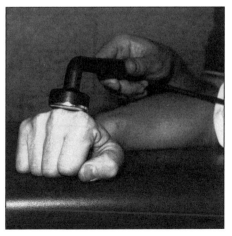

a   b

∎ **Figure 14.1** *(a)* Ultrasound heads of different sizes. Choose the ultrasound head that will give uniform contact with the body part. Dosage is determined for a treatment area that is two times the ERA (effective radiating area) of the sound head. *(b)* This ultrasound transducer does not provide complete contact with the treatment surface. A small transducer should be used, or underwater ultrasound should be performed.

APPLICATION OF ULTRASOUND

The most common method of applying ultrasound is by direct contact between the skin and the sound head. Ultrasound cannot be propagated through air, so there must be a coupling agent to provide air-free contact. The coupling medium should be inert, should transmit waves readily, and should contain no dissolved gases. Commercial gels or creams commonly are used.

DIRECT ULTRASOUND

Loss of consistent skin contact could result in an inconsistent treatment or damage to the crystal. Superficial heating of the sound head may indicate improper transmission. The sound head always should be kept moving, to minimize the chances of creating hot-spots. The pace should be about 3 to 4 cm/sec; faster movement results in a less than therapeutic effect. If the BNR is high, then the sound head must be moved faster to accommodate for the inconsistencies in the ultrasound beam. The BNR must be recorded on the machine or the transducer.

Instructions to the athlete should include information about the treatment and what is expected. Position the athlete comfortably and in a stretched position if increased range of motion is the goal. Mild warmth may be felt, but the athlete should immediately report any other sensation. Sharp pain may indicate periosteal irritation and burning.

Use the following rules for ultrasound application:

1. Keep the sound head moving at all times—check the speed.

2. Maintain full contact with the skin during the entire treatment. Keeping the sound head still can cause burning, and lifting it in the air can break the crystal or its housing. If keeping full contact is impossible, then a different sized sound head should be used or the indirect application is indicated.

3. If any sensation other than mild warmth is felt, the athlete should report it immediately. The speed of movement can be increased or the intensity must be decreased.

4. The athlete should not turn the machine on or determine the dosage for the ultrasound treatment.

INDIRECT ULTRASOUND

With indirect ultrasound, either water or a gel-filled bladder is used as the coupling agent. This method commonly is used for areas too small or irregular to maintain appropriate contact. When underwater ultrasound is used, both the sound head and the area to be treated are submerged in de-gassed, tepid water. Water is de-gassed by letting it sit for several hours before the treatment. With a gel-filled bladder, coupling gel must be placed on the skin to prevent an air interface.

The previous rules also apply in indirect or underwater ultrasound, except it is not necessary to have contact with the skin. The sound head should be held about 0.5 to 1.0 inch from the skin, and it must be moving. Any bubbles that form on the sound head or skin should be wiped off, because they can impede transmission into the tissues. The sound head should be held parallel to the tissues.

The dosage should be increased up to 0.5 W/cm^2 because of the energy dissipation in the water. The water temperature should be warm if a thermal effect is desired (see figure 14.2).

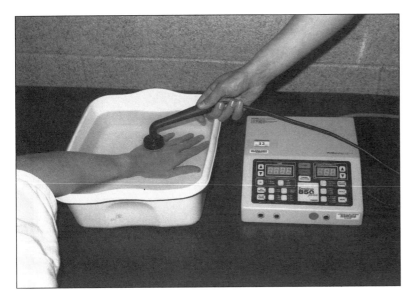

Figure 14.2 Indirect ultrasound. A container should be filled with water of the appropriate temperature and allowed to sit so that bubbles will dissipate. The ultrasound should be delivered by moving the sound head over the affected area. Increase intensity by 0.5 W/cm^2.

ULTRASOUND WITH ELECTRICAL STIMULATION

Because there is minimal perception of ultrasound energy during the treatment, ultrasound may be combined with electrical stimulation for pain modulation. This treatment combines the effects of the two modalities by connecting the units so that the electrical stimulation is emitted through the sound head. This method is useful in treating muscle spasms or local trigger points as well as providing massage effects.

The treatment time is determined by the ultrasound alone. Precautions for electrical stimulation also apply with this technique. Any current can be used if the units are equipped to be connected. Commonly, both high-voltage and low-voltage stimulators allow this treatment. A tetanizing frequency can be used, but the treatment may be more massage-like when a lower frequency stimulation in the 2 to 10 pps range is used.

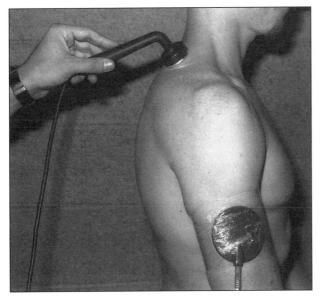

An adequate amount of conductive medium should be used. Mineral oil does not conduct electricity well and should not be used as a coupling agent.

Remember to keep the sound head moving, especially if the electrical stimulation must be adjusted. If two separate units are used, coincide the timers so the treatments end at the same time. Combination treatments should only be conducted with units that are designed for this purpose (see figure 14.3).

Figure 14.3 Electrical stimulation combined with ultrasound. The ultrasound head becomes the active electrode and the dispersive electrode should be securely fastened.

PHONOPHORESIS

Phonophoresis allows the application of molecules through the skin and into the superficial structures by using ultrasound. It is a painless and safe means of application of some medicines. The increase in cell membrane permeability caused by ultrasound promotes absorption of some medications.

Medications are commonly used substances including topical anti-inflammatory drugs. However, the medication must be prescribed by a physician. Always check if the athlete is allergic to any drug (e.g., salicylates). Some medications prevent the transmission of ultrasound. Generally, any thick cream cannot be used for phonophoresis. For example, hydrocortisone is a thick cream that blocks ultrasound transmission.

Because the amount of drug that penetrates intact skin is minimal, it may be advantageous for the medication to be in contact with the skin for a period longer than the ultrasound treatment. Use of an occlusive dressing has been suggested to keep the medication in place without dilution by the conductive medium. The medication and dressing should remain in place for at least 30 min and can remain on the skin after the treatment to promote further absorption. The substance is placed on the skin, and air bubbles are eliminated. More gel may be needed to provide adequate coupling. Ultrasound parameters should be consistent with the pathology.

Name_____   Date_____

Activities

1. Wrap tape around the outside of the transducer. Apply different types of gels and creams to the surface of the sound head. Turn up the intensity to see the output configuration of the machine. If no bubbles form, the cream blocks the ultrasound transmission. Note your findings here.

2. Place the sound head into a bucket of water. Wipe away all air bubbles that form. Turn the intensity up to 1.5 W/cm^2. Have a volunteer place a finger in the ultrasound beam and note any intensity changes here.

3. Find the BNR and the ERA on the ultrasound machine. Discuss how variations in ERA affect the treatment duration. How does BNR affect the treatment?

4. Using the following patient problems, determine intensities, durations, duty cycles, and frequencies of ultrasound application. Also note patient position.

    Case A: Your patient has an extension contracture in his left knee 10 weeks after an anterior cruciate ligament intra-articular reconstruction. His range of motion is limited to 95° of flexion.

    What adjunctive treatment would you recommend?

    Note the position you would choose, the area you would treat, and the dosage.

    Case B: A runner has plantar fasciitis that has prevented her from running for the last 4 weeks; she describes sharp pain on the medial aspect of the heel.

    Note the treatments you would recommend.

Case C: A patient has adhesive capsulitis of the shoulder. There have been improvements, but there is still decreased range of motion in external rotation.

Note the position that would best be used to treat this problem.

Case D: An athlete complains of bilateral pain in the lumbar region of the low back.

Describe this treatment with respect to duration, intensity, frequency, and choice of transducer size.

Case E: A 15-year-old soccer player has had subacute Achilles tendinitis for 3 weeks. There is decreased dorsiflexion.

What method would be most helpful in gaining range of motion?

Case F: A field hockey player has shinsplints. You have tried arch supports, stretching and strengthening of the leg muscles, and using ice after practice. You decide to try ultrasound for 10 treatments in a nonthermal manner.

What parameters are appropriate?

5. Demonstrate and note below a technique to increase range of motion using ultrasound.

LAB 15

Diathermy

Review material from chapter 9, pages 168 to 170 of the textbook, before you complete this lab.

OBJECTIVES

- You will understand the frequencies used for short-wave and microwave diathermy.

- You will understand when diathermy, rather than ultrasound, should be used for deep heat.

- You will understand contraindications and precautions for diathermy.

Diathermy is a deep heat modality that is not often used in sports medicine. There are precautions to diathermy, such as not using it over metal implants, but its advantages include the heating of large surfaces. Deep heat to the erector spinae muscles cannot be adequately delivered using ultrasound, and diathermy is an alternative treatment. Diathermy could be a good choice for deep heat in sports medicine because few athletes have large amounts of adipose tissue that insulates deeper tissues, blocking treatments. Additionally, short-wave diathermy is not reflected by the periosteum, making it a safer heating modality than ultrasound in some cases.

SHORT-WAVE AND MICROWAVE DIATHERMY

Short-wave and microwave diathermy uses the conversion of high-frequency electromagnetic energy to heat biological tissues. Diathermy is part of the electromagnetic spectrum and has properties of electromagnetic energy. Both short-wave diathermy and microwave diathermy are methods used to generate heat in superficial musculature. Diathermy also has been used in the pulsed mode on the theory that nonthermal energy will stimulate the activity of the cells and promote healing, much like nonthermal ultrasound. The electromagnetic fields generated within the injured tissues have been associated with decreased pain and swelling in double-blind studies. Other studies, however, are inconclusive and show no beneficial results with pulsed diathermy.

The Federal Communications Commission has designated several bands of frequencies for medical use. Although three frequencies of short-wave diathermy are available, the most commonly used short-wave frequency is 27.12 MHz with a wavelength of 11 m. This has the widest bandwidth and is the easiest to generate. Microwave diathermy has a single frequency of 2450 MHz.

Short-wave diathermy uses two types of electrode setups, the condenser (capacitive) or inductance (inductive) fields, to produce heat. The condenser field (e.g., air-space plates) uses the patient's body as a part of the circuit between the two conducting electrodes. Causing the molecules to vibrate in the tissues generates heat. The greatest heating occurs near the electrodes where the current density is greatest.

The inductance field places the patient in the electromagnetic field of the electrodes. The cable or hinged drum electrodes are used with the inductance fields. Heat is induced in superficial tissues and subsequently conducted to deeper tissues. The inductance coil has an alternating current passing through it. This current produces a magnetic field perpendicular to the coil, which induces eddy currents in the tissue. The eddy currents cause oscillation of molecules, which generates heat (see figure 15.1).

Diathermy can be used in athletic training to increase metabolism, cause vasodilation, and promote muscle relaxation. The advantages of using diathermy are that this treatment produces deeper heat than that obtained with hot packs and there is the ability to heat larger areas than with ultrasound.

The disadvantages of diathermy are the expense of the equipment, the inability to visualize the treatment area, and the possibility that high adiposity will result in burns. Diathermy should not be used with patients who are pregnant or who have infections, open epiphyses, pacemakers, metal implants (e.g., intra-uterine devices), malignancy, or obesity. Diathermy should not be used with very young or very old patients, due to the possibility of thermoregulatory compromise. It should not be used on ischemic areas, over the eyes or testes, or in the presence of perspiration or moist dressings. The diathermy unit should be 3 to 5 m away from electronic or magnetic equipment, such as computers, interferential units, or electrocardiogram devices. Finally, the patient should remove all metal objects, such as jewelry.

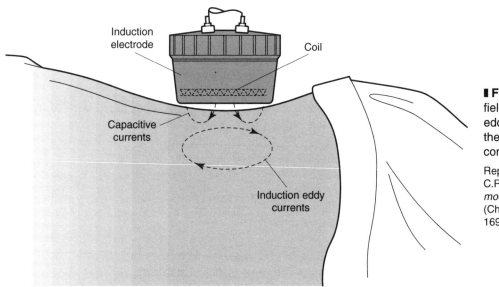

Figure 15.1 With magnetic field diathermy applicators, eddy currents are induced in the tissues having highest conductivity.

Reprinted, by permission, from C.R. Denegar, 2000, *Therapeutic modalities for athletic injuries* (Champaign, IL: Human Kinetics), 169.

APPLICATION OF DIATHERMY

Position the athlete comfortably on a table with no metal supports. All pillows with metal zippers and all jewelry in the treatment area should be removed. Drape the athlete to access the body part to be treated. Instruct the athlete to remain still throughout the treatment. Assess the treatment area for inflammation, skin irritations, and circulation. Apply a single layer of toweling on the treatment area to absorb any sweat that may accumulate during the treatment.

For an inductive treatment, place the drum with the enclosed coil parallel to the treatment area and in contact with the towel. For a capacitive treatment, position the plates parallel with the treatment area and about 2.5 to 8 cm away from the body.

Turn on the short-wave diathermy. Tell the athlete that he or she should only perceive warmth and if the treatment becomes hot, you should be alerted. Adjust the intensity and duration of treatment of the short-wave diathermy. Recheck the athlete after 5 min for excessive warmth, dripping sweat, or discomfort. When the treatment time is complete, turn the intensity dial to zero and remove the generator from the athlete. Assess the efficacy of the treatment and check the integrity of the skin.

Name_____   Date_____

Activities

1. Demonstrate and note below the proper application technique of diathermy. Use both the inductance and the capacitive methods for application.

2. With the following patient problems, discuss and note below when diathermy should be used for deep heat compared with ultrasound.
   - Bilateral paraspinal spasm without specific pathology to the spine.
   - Offensive lineman (280 lb) with a stiff shoulder.
   - Flexion contracture to 30° following a total knee replacement.
   - Tight quadriceps muscle before an isokinetic test.

LAB 16

Lumbar Traction

Review material from chapter 10, pages 184 to 192 of the textbook, before you complete this lab.

OBJECTIVES

- You will understand the techniques of lumbar traction.

- You will be able to describe different positions for traction.

- You will understand contraindications and precautions for traction.

SPINAL TRACTION

Spinal traction is the application of a distracting force to separate the vertebral joint surfaces. Traction can be applied manually or mechanically by using various protocols. The effects of spinal traction are to separate the vertebral bodies and facet joints, stretch the ligaments and facet joint capsules, and widen the intervertebral foramen. Traction also can straighten spinal curves and stretch spinal musculature when the traction force is increased. The angle of traction—flexion, extension, or side-bending—changes the location of greatest separation in the spine. The angle of traction can be altered by patient positioning or by adjusting the traction unit.

Spinal traction is indicated for the treatment of herniated nucleus pulposus with disc protrusion (the most common indication for traction). It has been demonstrated radiologically that traction can centralize the nucleus of the disc and may reduce a bulged disc. Reducing the bulge also can relieve pain of impinged nerve roots. However, the reduction is only temporary, and further management including exercise, posture correction, and education regarding proper body mechanics is imperative.

When the compressive pressures are relieved from the vertebral bodies, the intervertebral discs are allowed to imbibe fluid. This process can contribute to healing of the annular structure. However, if the duration of traction with large forces is excessive, the disc may draw too much fluid, resulting in increased pain.

Traction also is used to manage facet joint impingement or pain. Flexing the spine during traction causes the facet joints to open and relieve pressure on the intervertebral foramen. Traction can increase mobility in the facet joints and may interrupt the pain–spasm cycle to encourage resolution of symptoms. Again, traction will not cure these problems, and other treatments must be incorporated into the athlete's program.

CONTRAINDICATIONS TO TRACTION

Spinal traction should not be used with acute traumatic injury because it may aggravate inflammation. As the injury matures, traction may be incorporated, but the force should be applied gradually to an effective level. If there is increased pain after traction, reduce the forces or discontinue this treatment. There should never be pain during a traction treatment.

Spinal traction should not be used when there are structural deformities secondary to a tumor or infection. The athletic trainer should be aware of the possibility of vertebral artery obstruction with any cervical mobilization. If the athlete reports dizziness with cervical rotation, traction should not be used. Traction also is contraindicated in cases of instability or fracture.

Indications for Spinal Traction

- Herniated disc
- Nerve root syndromes
- Degenerative joint disease
- Joint hypomobility
- Pain relief and muscle spasms

Contraindications for Spinal Traction

- Acute strains or sprains
- Acute inflammation
- Joint hypermobility
- Pregnancy
- Rheumatoid arthritis
- Osteoporosis

TYPES OF SPINAL TRACTION

Spinal traction can be applied in several different ways. Manual, mechanical, intermittent, and auto-traction are some of the types of traction available.

MANUAL TRACTION

The clinician performs manual traction by using his or her hands to apply a force directly to the athlete. Because of the weight of the lower extremities, manual traction is used more commonly with cervical traction than with lumbar traction. The clinician grasps the head of the athlete, usually at the occiput and mandible, and pulls. Slow, intermittent forces should be applied with feedback from the athlete to determine the amount of pull necessary. Manual traction can be used in conjunction with mobilization techniques to increase range of motion. Because the forces can be monitored more easily and tailored to patient comfort, manual traction may be used before mechanical traction is implemented to determine if mechanical traction will be tolerated.

MECHANICAL TRACTION

Mechanical traction can be applied with a variety of techniques. Sustained (static) traction involves a constant pull for a certain amount of time. The only adjustment is made by taking up the slack as the athlete relaxes. Sustained traction is accomplished by commercial units, by hanging weights from the athlete's waist, or with positional traction in which body positioning creates the traction force. The duration of sustained traction is usually up to 30 min. Static traction is recommended for conditions with radicular symptoms.

INTERMITTENT MECHANICAL TRACTION

Intermittent mechanical traction is another form of spinal traction in which a commercial device is used to provide a consistent force that is applied and released according to a duty cycle. Lumbar traction can be applied intermittently and is most effective when a split table is used to decrease the frictional forces. The tractional force can be applied with any time sequence but is most commonly used at a 30-sec "on" time with 15 sec of rest. The traction force is reduced during the "off" time, but it is not eliminated. With this protocol, traction time should not exceed 10 min; therefore, total treatment time is generally about 15 to 20 min. Treatment time includes time for progressively increasing the force at the start of treatment and decreasing force at the end of treatment so that the compressive forces at the spine are reinstated gradually. Intermittent traction is indicated for hypomobile conditions.

APPLICATION OF TRACTION

The amount of force exerted in traction determines the amount of separation at the vertebral joints. However, this force always must be limited by symptoms or discomfort and should not cause pain during the treatment. To achieve traction, 50 to 100% of the body weight should be applied to the lumbar spine. Without a split table, lumbar traction forces must be greatly increased to be effective because it takes a force of one half the body weight to overcome frictional forces between the body and table. In initial treatments, low weights should be used to prevent counterproductive muscle spasm. Optimal pull initially is determined by trial and error, using the results of the evaluation and patient interaction as a guide. The force can be increased or decreased in subsequent treatments depending on the outcomes of the traction.

Relaxation of the spinal musculature is important for traction. Relaxation should be achieved before traction and can be enhanced with other modalities such as TENS, superficial heat, or ultrasound. To maintain relaxation after traction, the athlete should lie still for 5 to 10 min without the pull. This allows the normal forces to be re-established and decreases the chance of reaggravating a facet joint. In addition, the athlete should avoid twisting the spine as he or she gets off the table and should avoid sudden weight bearing.

The athlete can be either supine (see figure 16.1) or prone according to comfort, but the degree of spinal flexion or extension during traction is determined by the condition being treated. Spinal flexion is appropriate for facet hypomobility and narrowed intervertebral foramen problems, whereas extension is recommended for discogenic symptoms. Relaxation and comfort are critical considerations for effective traction application.

The athlete should wear minimal clothing to ensure belt-to-skin contact and to prevent the belts from slipping. Position the harnesses appropriately on the table. The edge of the thoracic belt should be at the split in the table with the pelvic harness overlapping so that it will extend above the iliac crest. Secure the pelvic belt first such that the iliac crest lies midway in the harness. Secure the thoracic belt so that it rests on the lower aspect of the rib cage. All belts should be secured snugly! You can place a towel under the buckles for comfort.

Place a stool underneath the athlete's legs to enhance comfort in the supine position. Attach the thoracic harness at the top of the table to provide the counter-traction. Attach the pelvic harness to the traction unit. A spreader bar may be used but generally is not required except for large patients. Provide a safety switch that will allow the athlete to discontinue the treatment if necessary.

Set the "off" cycle and "on" cycle poundage. The "off" cycle poundage is generally set at 50% of the maximum setting. The "on" cycle poundage is determined by the athlete's tolerance so that there is no discomfort and neurological symptoms are not exacerbated. Generally, a minimum of 25% of the athlete's body weight is used initially. Treatment time and poundage are progressed with subsequent treatment sessions as tolerance is shown.

The hold time is determined by the type of traction chosen. Intermittent traction is usually applied for 30 sec and released for 15 sec. The treatment duration is set initially for approximately 5 min and progresses to a maximum of 10 min once the maximal tension has been established. Static traction is applied from 10 to 30 min. This does not include the progression or regression time it takes to reach or decline from the desired poundage. Changes in poundage should be gradual to promote relaxation.

After the unit has cycled two to three times, release the table lock. This should be done during the rest phase while the clinician stabilizes the table to prevent jerking. The delay is to take the

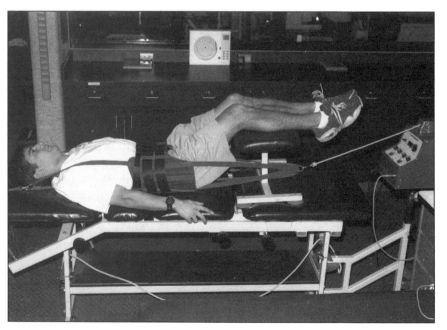

∎ **Figure 16.1** Mechanical traction. The athlete is supine with the legs supported and the hips and knees flexed.

"slack" out of the setup. The treatment poundage is increased by 10% over the next five successive cycles.

Following the treatment, the table is locked and the harnesses are released. The athlete should lie on the table for the next 5 to 10 min to allow the tissues to approximate gradually. Exercise can be performed after traction.

PRONE TRACTION

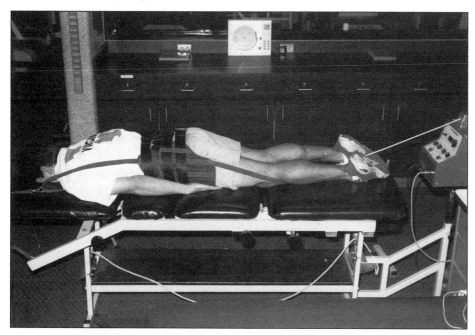

Prone traction is used when extension of the spine is emphasized. No radiating symptoms should be present in the prone position and the athlete should be able to lie prone without pain. The belts are put on while the athlete is standing, and the buckles should be in the back (see figure 16.2).

■ **Figure 16.2** Prone traction. The harness is applied to the athlete with the buckles on the back. The athlete lies prone and the traction is applied so that the spine is in greater extension than it is in supine traction.

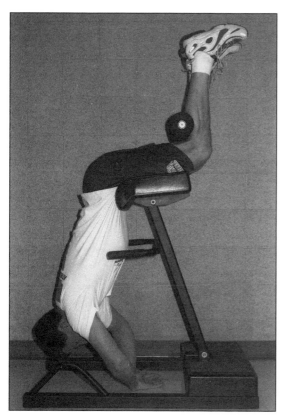

AUTO-TRACTION

When a traction table is not available, auto-traction using gravity may be performed. It is imperative that the athlete can tolerate an upside-down position. An auto-traction device can be used, or the athlete can suspend himself or herself from a back hyperextension machine.

The athlete simply holds on with the legs and attempts to relax the spine as much as possible. Because of the position, short intervals (less than 1 min) are used at first, and intervals are increased as the athlete feels comfortable (see figure 16.3).

■ **Figure 16.3** Auto-traction. The athlete places him- or herself into the device and slowly turns upside down. The athlete is encouraged to relax during treatment.

Name_____ Date_____

Activities

1. Practice setting up a partner on lumbar traction. Follow the procedure to ensure safety. Use the prone or supine position.

2. Using the following patient problems, demonstrate and discuss the traction technique to use. Note below the position, method, and weights to be used in the initial treatment and in subsequent treatments.

   Case A: A 145-lb soccer goal-keeper has minimal back pain but describes numbness along the back of the leg and into the heel. She is unable to do a single-leg calf raise on the affected side.

   Case B: A 215-lb athlete reports to the athletic training room with a lateral shift to the right and is unable to stand erect without pain.

   If manual traction increases pain, should mechanical traction be used as a treatment?

   Case C: A 230-lb football player had a collision with another player and has pain, spasm, and limitation in all spine motions. There are minor discogenic symptoms.

   Case D: A 136-lb wrestler has low back pain. He has a forward-flexed posture (not caused by pain) and a flat lumbar spine. Extension relieves his pain.

LAB 17

Cervical Traction

Review material from chapter 10, pages 184 to 192 of the textbook, before you complete this lab.

OBJECTIVES

- You will understand the principles of cervical traction as part of a comprehensive rehabilitation program.

- You will understand various methods of cervical traction.

- You will understand the implications of the angle of pull and the weight progression.

- You will understand the indications and contra-indications of cervical traction.

The philosophy of treatment and theories of cervical traction are the same as those for lumbar traction, except the weights are much lower. The effects on the discs, vertebral joint structures, and paraspinal musculature are similar with lumbar and cervical traction.

VERTEBRAL ARTERY TEST

Before any manipulation of the cervical spine, either with mechanical or manual traction, the circulatory status should be ascertained. A bony anomaly may cause pressure on the vertebral artery, which is responsible for the blood supply to the brain. Clear the vertebral artery by having the patient rotate his or her head as far as possible in one direction and then the other. Hold the position of maximal rotation for at least 15 sec. If the patient becomes dizzy or nauseated, do not perform any mechanical therapies on the neck.

TRACTION POSITION

Patient comfort is of utmost importance, because a comfortable position will cause the greatest relaxation and therefore the most therapeutic treatment. The relative degree of flexion or extension, however, can affect which surfaces of the vertebrae are separated the most effectively. Spinal flexion results in greater separation of the posterior structures, and extension causes greatest separation of the anterior structures. The posterior structures include the facet joints and the intervertebral foramen, whereas the anterior structures are the vertebral bodies and disks. With cervical traction, more flexion also causes a greater force to be directed at the lower cervical region, whereas a neutral or slightly extended position causes more force at the upper cervical region. An angle of 24° is recommended for maximal posterior elongation.

MECHANICAL CERVICAL TRACTION

The athlete should be in a supine position for cervical traction. The angle of traction should be 5 to 20° of flexion unless a greater degree of flexion is more comfortable. A pillow can be placed underneath the knees and behind the neck to enhance comfort. A head halter is attached to the mandible and to the occiput (see figure 17.1). The degree of cervical flexion is adjusted by tightening the straps to the occiput where most of the pull should be directed. The halter is attached to the traction unit by using a spreader bar. Take care not to exert too much pressure on the temporomandibular joint. If a Saunders traction device is used, do not overly tighten the forehead strap. The occiput device should fit snugly and not slide during the treatment. The Saunders device allows less pressure to the mandible, which can avoid temporomandibular joint aggravation. Provide the athlete with the safety shutoff switch.

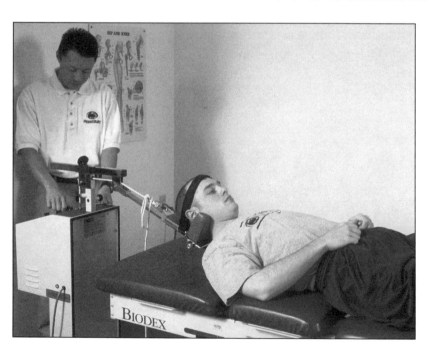

▌Figure 17.1   Cervical traction with Saunder's device.

Adjust the on/off cycle when using intermittent traction. Gradually increase the poundage to the desired amount. Some units provide a safety toggle that will not allow more than 40 lb of cervical traction unless engaged. More weight may be needed for larger athletes such as football players, although this is unusual. Following the treatment, the athlete should remain supine for 5 to 10 min. Gradual therapeutic exercise can be initiated at this time.

Do not leave the patient alone during traction. Reassess the patient after 5 min and make adjustments if necessary. It is better to build up to an effective traction force over several treatments, because too great a force can increase pain and spasm even hours after the treatment has ended. Instruct the patient to stop the force or alert you if there is increased pain or any peripheralization of symptoms.

MANUAL TRACTION/DISTRACTION

Manual distraction of the cervical spine is easier than distraction of the lumbar spine because the weight of the head is generally only 8 to 10 lb. Sit or stand at the end of a treatment table with the patient's head in your hands. Your position is determined by the height of the table. Good body position—standing close to the athlete's head without bending over—is essential to minimize your fatigue and prevent injury. Grasp the head with both hands under the occipital process and gently pull. Emphasize axial extension and make sure the patient is relaxed (see figure 17.2).

The degree of spinal flexion can be manipulated to direct the force to the lower cervical spine or upper thoracic vertebrae. Cycle the traction for 30 to 40 sec, and then release. The individual mobility in the anteroposterior direction of each spinous process can be assessed in this position. Likewise, varying degrees of lateral side bending and opposite rotation stress the facet joints.

The benefit of manual traction is that the clinician is sensitive to the degree of relaxation and amount of pain with the treatment and can adjust the amount of pull accordingly. The force also can be directed at different joints throughout the treatment. A disadvantage, however, is that the amount of traction is limited by the clinician's strength and fatigue. A long, sustained force, which might be necessary to centralize a herniation, is not possible. Furthermore, the treatment demands one-on-one time, which may not be possible in a busy athletic training room.

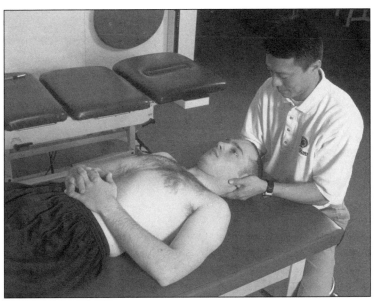

▌Figure 17.2
Manual cervical traction.

OVER-THE-DOOR TRACTION UNITS

Over-the-door cervical traction units are designed for home use. They are inexpensive and easy to set up, and the apparatus uses the weight of water over a pulley to elicit the traction force. Patients who have recurrent neck pain should consider purchasing a home unit. These units can be used for static traction only, because they cannot cycle. A disadvantage of this therapy is that the patient must sit and therefore the weight of the head has to be unloaded before the joints are distracted. The patient should be educated about weight, posture, and the duration and frequency of the treatment.

WEIGHT PROGRESSION

Initial cervical traction weights generally are estimated by the patient's tolerance to manual traction. If manual traction is well tolerated, then mechanical traction can be started. Note that the weights described here are for supine traction in which the weight of the head has been minimized. For sitting traction, 5 to 10 lb is generally added. In the early stages, begin with a 5- to 10-min treatment with 7 to 15 lb, depending on the size of the athlete. If this treatment is well tolerated, then gradually increase the time to 20 to 30 min. Remember that symptoms may return several hours after the end of the treatment. The weight eventually can be increased up to 20 to 40 lb.

CONTRAINDICATIONS TO CERVICAL TRACTION

Cervical traction should not be done with patients who have rheumatoid arthritis, Marfan's syndrome, or Down's syndrome (may have instability at C1/2). Cervical traction should not be used in acute inflammation. You can feel for heat, swelling, or other acute signs of inflammation or lymph adenopathy. Use caution with patients who have pain in the temporomandibular joint unless you are using a head holder that does not compress the jaw.

Name_____ Date_____

Discussion Question

1. Discuss and note when cervical traction, including manual traction, can be used as part of a rehabilitation program.

Activities

1. Demonstrate the proper application technique of cervical traction. Discuss and note below the consequences of varying degrees of spinal flexion during the treatment.

2. Practice a vertebral artery test. Practice manual traction on a partner. Note the differences in the location of distraction when different positions are used.

3. Discuss the treatment of cervical traction with the following case study. Note precautions, the position of traction, and the weight progression.

Case A: A 37-year-old retired football player (210 lb) has recurrent neck pain. There is generally no provocative incident, but at times he wakes up unable to turn his head to the right side due to pain and stiffness. Evaluation reveals good posture but an overdevelopment of the anterior shoulder musculature. Mild weakness is noted in the right thumb opposition. There is no sensory deficit or paresthesia. The upper thoracic region has active trigger points on the right side that are painful to palpation. Active range of motion in the cervical spine demonstrates a 50% decrease in right rotation, and right side-bending also is limited by pain. Flexion and extension are normal. Manual cervical assessment demonstrates pain with anteroposterior glide of T1 through C2 and restriction in motion at C5/C6. Manual distraction relieves pain.

Describe the treatment for this patient and note some options for this recurring problem.

LAB 18

Intermittent Compression

Review material from chapter 10, pages 192 to 193 of the textbook, before you complete this lab.

OBJECTIVES

- You will be able to measure edema and establish methods of treatment.

- You will understand the use of intermittent compression in conjunction with elevation and muscle pumping to decrease edema.

- You will understand contraindications and precautions for intermittent compression.

INTERMITTENT PNEUMATIC COMPRESSION DEVICES

Intermittent pneumatic compression devices such as Jobst or Pression effectively reduce peripheral edema. They can be used in conjunction with elevation or in some cases with cooling to help minimize inflammation and edema accumulation with acute injuries. As the injury matures and pitting edema remains, these devices also can contribute to the reabsorption of the extravasated fluid and inflammatory by-products by augmenting lymphatic function.

Tissue trauma results in edema as blood vessel damage and inflammatory reactions allow whole blood and plasma to leak into the interstitial space. The extent of edema depends on the amount of vessel damage and the clotting response that is activated immediately. Edema can continue to develop in the first 24 to 48 h in acute inflammation when blood flow and vessel permeability are increased. Leakage of plasma proteins disrupts the osmotic pressures between the intravascular region and the interstitium. The increased interstitial osmotic pressure draws more fluid out of the capillaries. Although much of this waste can be reabsorbed as healing transpires, plasma proteins, because of their large size, must be taken up by the lymphatics. Within limits, lymph action increases as interstitial pressures increase; the pressure widens the junctions between cells (valves), allowing the reabsorption of larger particles. Muscle pumping and intrinsic rhythmical contractions propel the fluid back to the heart, where it can be metabolized.

The treatment of edema should incorporate any agent that changes the relative pressures at the capillary wall. Elevation and external compression provide an additional force that inhibits leakage of fluid out of the capillary and aids reabsorption. Using a pneumatic appliance that fits entirely around the swollen extremity provides uniform pressure for this purpose. Some units use circulating freon or ice-water to simultaneously provide the benefits of cold therapy (50-75° F). Compression should be maintained throughout the day by using a compression bandage, wrap, or compression stocking. Wraps should be comfortable and should cover the area thoroughly with even pressure. Wrinkles in the wraps should be minimized, because they cause additional pressure or constriction.

Intermittent compression is indicated whenever there is traumatic edema or venous insufficiency. Intermittent compression should not be used if there is any sign of an infection or in the presence of thrombophlebitis. This therapy should not be used if there is an obstruction of the lymphatics or if the patient has a history of congestive heart failure.

APPLICATION

Place the athlete in a position so that the injured structure is elevated above the level of the heart. Measure the girth of the area before and after treatment to document the effectiveness of the treatment. Place a cotton stocking or stockinet on the extremity to absorb perspiration and to add comfort (minimize wrinkles in the stocking or stockinet). Put the extremity in the pneumatic device and connect the air delivery tube. The athlete should be comfortable.

Completely loosen the pressure control knobs to prevent overpressurization. Turn the power on, keeping the off-cycle on the zero position to provide continuous pressure while determining the appropriate pressure. Increase the pressure while observing the pressure gauge. Suggested operating pressures are 40 to 60 mm Hg for the upper extremity and 60 to 100 mm Hg for the lower extremity. The pressure should be tolerable, and the athlete should not feel pulsations, pain, or paresthesia in the extremity.

Set the duty cycle; a 90-sec "on" time and 30-sec "off" time (a 3:1 on/off cycle) is usually suggested. The total treatment time varies from 20 min to 1 hr or even longer. The treatments can be repeated twice a day. During the rest phase, active motion in a pain-free range can be performed to enhance edema resorption.

Following treatment, wrinkles may appear on the skin. These wrinkles are of no consequence and usually disappear 20 to 30 min after treatment is discontinued. Posttreatment girth measurements are advised. An elastic wrap should be applied after the treatment to help sustain the reduction. Intermittent compression can be continued as long as pre- and posttreatment girth measurements indicate that progress is being made (see figure 18.1).

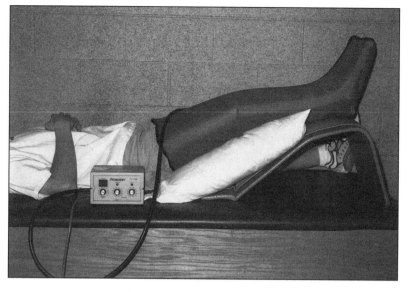

❚ Figure 18.1 Intermittent compression. The appropriate appliance should be used to encompass the edematous area. The pressure and duty cycle should be set and the limb comfortably elevated.

ELASTIC WRAPS

Wraps should be used whenever edema or effusion is present. The athlete should wear some type of compression at all times, although the wrap should be loosened at night. Take care to wrap evenly with firm pressure and to overlap by one half the width of the wrap; use spirals because circumferential wrapping can cause too much constriction. Avoid "windows", or gaps, in which edema can accumulate, and avoid wrinkles in the wrap that add compression. Felt pads can add compression at contusion sites or around bony prominences such as the malleoli of the ankle. Always encourage elevation! Show the athlete how to rewrap the part more loosely if there is throbbing or aching (see figure 18.2).

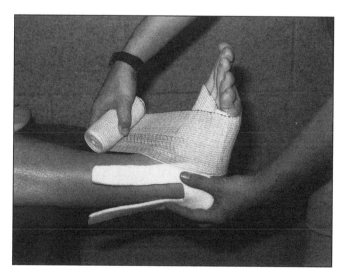

a

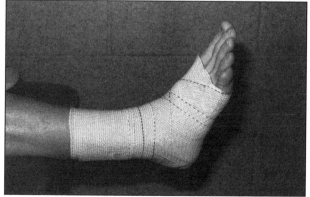

b

❚ Figure 18.2 Elastic wrap. Begin wrapping at the distal aspect and wrap proximally *(a)*. Use a horseshoe or pad so that even compression occurs around bony prominences *(b)*.

ANTIEMBOLISM STOCKINGS

Another method of applying compression to the lower extremity is to use antiembolism stockings. This method eliminates the need to teach the athlete how to apply an elastic wrap. The hose should be tight but not constrictive, and wrinkles should be avoided (see figure 18.3).

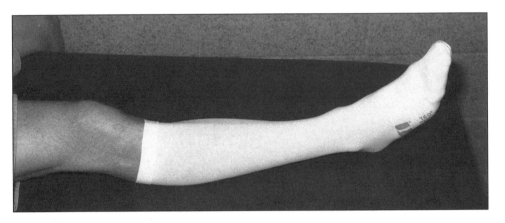

▮ Figure 18.3   Antiembolism stocking. Compression is applied evenly along the entire limb.

Name_____ Date_____

Activities

1. In groups, practice setting up an intermittent compression treatment with an ankle, knee, or hand. Note the pressures tolerated prior to perceived pulsations in the upper extremity compared with the lower extremity. Note the difficulty in elevating the limb during the treatment for the upper extremity.

2. Set up the intermittent compression device with an ice pack. What alterations should be made in the treatment? Note the pressures that are tolerated.

3. Practice wrapping the ankle, knee, elbow, and wrist with elastic bandages. Try to overlap by one half the width of the wrap on each turn and angle the wrap so that circumferential pressure is not applied. Make sure the wrap stays in place with normal activity. Use felt pads to increase pressure around bony prominences.

LAB 19

Massage

Review material from chapter 13, pages 177 to 178 of the textbook, before you complete this lab.

OBJECTIVES

- You will understand the principles of soft-tissue massage and how it is used in rehabilitation.

- You will understand the types of massage, including Hoffa massage, the cross-fiber friction massage, scar tissue mobilization, and Shiatsu acupressure.

Massage has been used in many forms for more than 3000 years. Massage currently is used as a relaxation modality, to gain range of motion, to mobilize scar tissue, and to increase blood flow. Massage can decrease pain and muscle spasm, improve circulation, facilitate healing, restore joint mobility, and enhance the removal of metabolites and lactic acid from muscle. In recent years a trend in manual therapies has brought massage back into the medical world. However, a medical society driven by insurance companies has scrutinized these manual procedures.

Massage therapy includes many different strokes. The four strokes commonly used in sports massage are effleurage, petrissage, kneading, and friction. These strokes offer a variety of effects and benefits.

EFFLEURAGE

Effleurage is slow, rhythmic, stroking hand movements with the hand molded to the skin throughout the stroke. Effleurage runs from the distal aspect of the tissue's long axis to the proximal end. The stroke is essentially a sliding motion over the skin. Sliding with a gradual compression reduces muscle tone and creates a general relaxation. More firm strokes can accelerate blood flow and lymph flow and can improve venous return. This stroke also can prepare an athlete for performance. Rapid strokes actually increase muscle tone and improve the athlete's level of readiness.

PETRISSAGE

Petrissage is a more vigorous massage stroke that is often associated with the Swedish massage for stress relief. Petrissage consists of folding, lifting, and rolling the subcutaneous and muscle tissue against the underlying tissue. This stroke is effective for stretching contracted and adhered tissue and helps to relieve muscle spasm. Petrissage also promotes the flow of blood and lymph and is effective in mobilizing pitting edema.

KNEADING

Kneading consists of slow circular compression of the soft tissue against the underlying bone. This stroke is applied with graded pressure as the clinician moves proximally. Kneading promotes fluid movement and loosens connective tissue shortened by scarring. This technique is effective for resolving trigger points.

FRICTION

Friction massage is an accurate, penetrating pressure applied through the fingers. There are two common types of friction massage: circular and transverse. Friction massage is often uncomfortable, and it causes a mild tissue-inflammatory reaction. Friction massage is especially useful in treating adhered soft tissue because collagen fiber alignment responds to imposed stress during the remodeling phase of inflammation.

The time required for massage is one of its biggest drawbacks. Like other modalities, massage may be an appropriate choice to treat the problem. However, athletic trainers may need to prioritize their treatments for therapeutic purposes rather than for the relaxation effects of massage.

PROCEDURE

1. A complete knowledge of the anatomical structures is important in all massage treatments.

2. The application of pressure is determined by the degree of inflammation and the type of tissue to be massaged. Pain should always be used as a guide and the pressure should be decreased appropriately. The clinician should position himself or herself with good body mechanics to prevent fatigue. For a general massage, the pressure should be delivered with the all parts of the hand and should be adjusted for the contours of the athlete's body.

3. An edematous extremity should be elevated during the massage to promote venous and lymph return.

4. The proximal aspect of a limb should be massaged first if there is edema. This minimizes the resistance in the lymph channels and enhances the resolution of edema in the distal part. This technique is termed *uncorking*.

5. The athlete should relax as much as possible, and the massage should not be painful. Furthermore, force should not be excessive enough to cause ecchymosis or discoloration after a massage.

6. An adequate amount of lubricant should be used to allow the hands to glide smoothly along the skin surface. More lubricant is necessary if the athlete has an excessive amount of body hair. Many commercially produced massage creams are available. These creams are manufactured to minimize absorption and drying during the massage while providing an appropriate amount of viscosity.

7. Strokes should overlap and should primarily be in a proximal direction to promote lymph absorption. Return strokes should have less pressure.

8. Bony prominences should be avoided (see figure 19.1).

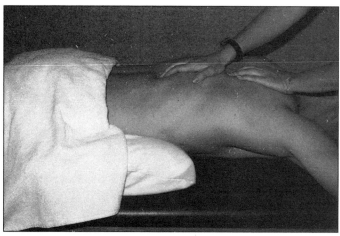

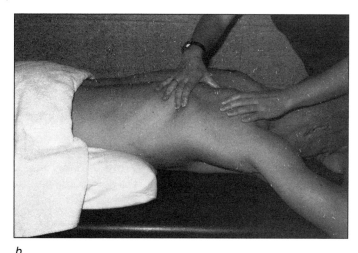

Figure 19.1 Massage. The area to be massaged should be relaxed, comfortable, and, if the area is swollen, elevated. *(a)* Effleurage: long strokes with gentle presure are applied along the area of massage. *(b)* Petrissage: specific areas are kneaded and squeezed with deeper pressure.

TYPES OF MASSAGE

Different types of massage can be used depending on the goal of the treatment. The types of massage include the general, or Hoffa, massage, cross-fiber friction massage, scar tissue mobilization, and Shiatsu acupressure.

HOFFA TECHNIQUE: CLASSIC MASSAGE

Long, light effleurage strokes are used at the beginning and end of the massage. The strokes are performed with the entire hand, which should be relaxed so that it conforms to the contours of the athlete's body. Strokes should move along the "grain" of the muscle fibers.

After several effleurage strokes, petrissage is performed. The full surface of both hands is used in a motion similar to kneading dough. The muscles are grasped and squeezed between the fingers, thumb, and palm of the hand and are lifted in a continuous alternating motion. Although this technique can be used on almost any body part with practice, it is best performed over areas of the body that have more soft tissue mass such as the hamstrings, gluteal area, paraspinals, or shoulders.

Tapotement is a percussion technique in which the therapist's hands are moved in a rapid and rhythmic pounding motion over the athlete's body. The hands may be relaxed, cupped, or held in a loose fist. Relaxed hands are held so that the thumb is pointing up and the ulnar side of the palm touches the athlete; this makes for a chopping motion. Cupped hands are held so that the proximal part of the palm, the ulnar side of the palm, the distal portion of the fingers, and the thumb touch the athlete and the middle portion of the palm forms a cup. This technique makes for a more gentle and less specific tapotement because the force is more distributed. Fists are used when more pressure and precision are desired. The most important things to remember are to avoid bony prominences and the area over the kidneys on the lower back and to keep the wrists relaxed at all times. If the wrists become stiff, the therapist risks self-injury as well as injury to the athlete. The massage generally ends with several strokes of effleurage.

CROSS-FIBER FRICTION

This technique is used to reduce adhesions in muscles. Adhesions are areas where the muscle or fascia has become plastered together so that it is tight and knotty or ropy. Adhesions can occur from injuries where scar tissue has been laid down, such as muscle and ligament pulls and strains, deep contusions, overuse, and surgery. Cross-fiber friction usually is performed with the pads of the thumbs and consists of small back-and-forth movements that go across the grain of the muscle or tendon. The amount of pressure used is determined in part by the age of the injury and in part by the comfort of the athlete. Cross-fiber friction is not indicated in acute injuries, and light work may be done on subacute injuries such as swelling reduction in an ankle sprain. In chronic injuries, the amount of pressure used is based on the athlete's pain tolerance.

SCAR-TISSUE MOBILIZATION

After a surgical procedure, the incision goes through changes that continue to adapt for up to 1 year. The scar heals with all tissue layers connected in a disorganized fashion. The skin should move freely over the soft tissue and the soft tissue should be free from the bone. This is often not the case after surgery, and the skin and soft tissue can reduce joint mobility.

The force of a scar-tissue mobilization should be a shearing motion. Do not use lubrication because your fingers should stick to the patient's skin. Dycem is a commercial product that can be used to improve adherence to the patient's skin. Transverse motion is used to move individual tissue layers. The scar can be moved in all directions, although the scar should not be pulled apart because this may stress the newly healing tissue and widen the scar. The scar should eventually be free from the underlying tissues.

Scar tissue mobilization may begin 2 to 3 weeks after surgery, focusing on the tissues surrounding the wound. Pressure should be mild but should increase as the scar matures and strengthens. At 6 weeks, aggressive scar-tissue mobilization is usually well tolerated (see figure 19.2).

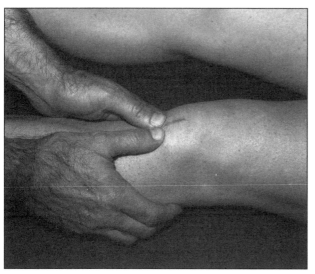 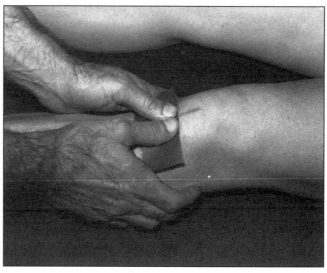

a   *b*

∎ Figure 19.2   Scar-tissue mobilization. Pressure to the skin is applied to free underlying structures *(a)*. Dycem is used to keep the clinician's fingers from slipping on the patient's skin *(b)*.

ACUPRESSURE (SHIATSU)

This technique, also sometimes called neuromuscular therapy, focuses on release of trigger points in muscles. Trigger points are relatively small areas of tension or spasm that build up in the body of muscles, often in high-stress areas. A trigger point can be very painful and can cause referred pain as well as increased tension in the rest of the muscle and even surrounding muscles. Release of a trigger point can relax an entire muscle or area of the body. Certain points in the body (acupressure points) are permanent trigger points and have specific areas of pain referral as well as those caused by vigorous athletic activity and daily stress. A trigger point may be found by stroking the muscle belly with the thumbs until a distinct area of tightness is found. To release the trigger point, direct pressure is applied by using one or both thumbs. A good way to gauge when a release has occurred is to have the athlete rate the pain on a scale of 1 to 10; when the athlete reaches 7, hold the point until the pain level has decreased to a 3 or 4. Anything above a 7 will be too painful for the athlete to relax. Often the trigger point will not completely release right away, and several of these releases must be used in a session. It is best to give a 1- or 2-min break to the area between releases, so that the body's natural endorphins are not stimulated.

Name_____ Date_____

Discussion Questions

1. Determine and note below when massage can be used to promote recovery and when aggressive massage may be contraindicated.

2. Discuss and note below what type of massage techniques or strokes should be used
   - Pre-event

   - Postevent

   - During/in-between events

   - During training

Activities

1. Demonstrate the proper application technique of massage.
2. Demonstrate and distinguish various types of massage and soft-tissue mobilization techniques.

LAB 20

Biofeedback

Review material from chapter 12, pages 208 to 213 of the textbook, before you complete this lab.

OBJECTIVES

- You will understand the uses of biofeedback in re-habilitation.

- You will be able use either biofeedback or neuro-muscular stimulation (see lab 10) for muscle re-education.

- You will be able to use biofeedback to inhibit muscle function and promote relaxation.

Biofeedback is the technique of revealing normal or abnormal characteristics of internal physiological events (muscular, visceral) in the form of auditory or visual signals. By learning to manipulate the displayed signals, the person is able to influence these involuntary or previously uncontrolled physiological events. None of the instruments "do" anything to the patient; they only give information about the events taking place in the patient's body. Each instrument acts as an external mirror for the internal state. Biofeedback training is an active treatment: the patient has full control of what is happening, and only he or she can affect results.

There is no guarantee that biofeedback training will help every patient, just as medications have different effects on different people. The goal is for the person to be able to volitionally control physiological events.

Methods of using feedback to reinforce behavior or activity include electromyography (EMG), electrocardiogram, electroencephalogram, or any tool that will reveal information about the body (e.g., a thermometer). Classically, these tools have been used in psychology to reduce tension and relieve stress. In athletic training, EMG is used to provide information about the muscle. In general, the tool must be sensitive enough to measure change.

EMG BIOFEEDBACK

EMG biofeedback can be contrasted with diagnostic EMG, in which the function of the peripheral nerves is being tested. With diagnostic EMG, usually needle electrodes are placed into the muscle supplied by a specific nerve. Both the amplitude and the waveform of the muscle's electrical discharge are measured. Neuropathies can be diagnosed, and nerve regeneration can be measured in this manner.

The voltage that is generated by the EMG is picked up by the electrodes either below the skin (needle electrodes) or on the skin (surface electrodes). Compared to needle electrodes, surface electrodes are less sensitive because of the electrical impedance or resistance of the skin. Surface electrodes require skin preparation to lower the skin resistance as much as possible, but skin preparation does not eliminate the resistance, which is more important when the microvoltage is to be quantified. A true measure of the voltage requires needle electrodes. In addition, the placement of the surface electrode will change the results because variations in cutaneous thickness will affect the impedance. The proximity to motor units also can vary results with surface electrodes.

COMPONENTS OF AN EMG

Amplifier, feedback method, gain, and threshold to signal are all components of an EMG. These parameters allow the clinician to adjust the EMG so that each treatment is individualized. Some EMGs have more than one channel, which increases their versatility, and the device may be connected to a computer to save the parameters and results of the treatment.

Amplifier

The amplifier magnifies the electrical signal produced by the voltage of action potential of the motor unit firing. The electrical impulse travels through the nerve and onto a muscle fiber. As the electrochemical discharge takes place, a measurable voltage occurs, usually in the microvolts (one millionth of a volt). The more motor units that are firing, the greater the total voltage.

Feedback Method

The method of informing the patient or athlete about the status of the contraction can be either an audio or visual signal. The audio signal is usually a beep, whereas the visual feedback may be a series of flashing lights, a meter, or a graph on a computer screen.

Gain

The gain is an adjustable parameter that affects the sensitivity of machine to electrical signal. Adjustments must be made so that the machine will be sensitive enough to indicate the response in the early stages of training and not so sensitive that large changes cannot be measured. The gain affects the scale of the EMG and is usually in multiples of the original scale. For instance, if the scale measures 10 to 50 μV, the gain will make the scale 20 to 100 (2$\times$) or 30 to 150 (3$\times$) or even 100 to 500 (10$\times$).

Another way to think of gain is to compare it with measurements of weight. To weigh infants, a scale must be sensitive enough to measure ounces so that progress can be documented. For adults, the scale must have a range higher than the weight of the subject; otherwise, you cannot obtain an accurate weight.

Threshold to Signal

The threshold to signal is another adjustable feature of the biofeedback unit. This parameter is the voltage that the athlete must overcome to produce the auditory or visual signal. The threshold and gain should be adjusted so that the athlete is continually stressed to improve.

USES OF BIOFEEDBACK

Biofeedback is used in rehabilitation for muscle re-education, to enhance the effectiveness of contracting a specific muscle over another, or to influence the relative activity of a specific muscle during a functional activity.

Biofeedback is used for muscle reeducation by overcoming the reflex inhibition following injury or surgery. Proprioception is lost with injury, and the athlete cannot perceive the muscle contraction. Biofeedback helps to reinforce the contraction so that muscle function can be relearned. Ultimately, there is improvement in the force development capacity of a muscle by coordinating motor units.

Biofeedback is used to preferentially improve the contraction of one muscle over another. For example, the athlete can be taught to isolate the contraction of the vastus medialis in quadriceps exercise to influence patellar tracking. Biofeedback can be used to induce relaxation by reinforcing a decrease in electrical activity.

Finally, biofeedback is used to teach the proper technique of therapeutic exercise. For example, the athlete is taught a functional activity such as raising the arm. Biofeedback can be used on the lower trapezius muscle to indicate whether this muscle is properly used to stabilize the scapula during the activity. Another example would be to monitor the activity of the quads during heel-strike. This technique is especially helpful if there is an extensor lag.

TECHNIQUE FOR KNEE REHABILITATION

Place electrodes on the vastus medialis, parallel to the muscle fibers. Gel may be needed to reduce the skin impedance. Initially, use a low threshold. The sensitivity should be in its highest position so that minimal activity will produce the desired response.

Give verbal cues to elicit a quadriceps isometric contraction. For patellofemoral problems, the knee should be in terminal extension. Some anterior cruciate ligament protocols may require the knee to be flexed to 30°, and a quad/hamstring cocontraction may be necessary. Biofeedback can be used throughout the exercise session to reinforce the quadriceps activity.

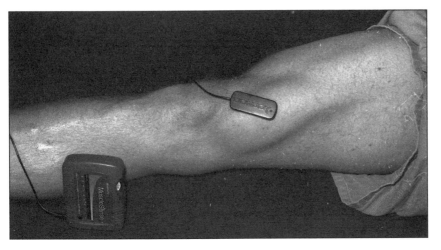

■ Figure 20.1 EMG biofeedback for vastus medialis obliquus. Skin is prepared and electrodes (all three are contained within a strip) are placed in parallel to the muscle fibers.

As the patient improves, adjust the threshold and sensitivity so that a stronger contraction will be necessary to elicit the EMG response. Electrode placement affects the EMG response, so changes from one treatment session to another may not correlate exactly with changes in muscle function. Increases in the gain and sensitivity will indicate improved muscle control (see figure 20.1).

IMPROVING RANGE OF MOTION

Tell the athlete to relax. Relaxation is indicated by a "quiet" EMG. Set the sensitivity so that a minimal contraction elicits feedback. Use a similar electrode placement or place the electrodes more generally on the quadriceps muscle. The patient should concentrate on relaxation and fluctuations of the feedback. The goal is to reduce the activity of the muscle to be stretched.

Passively move the limb to the end of the range; usually there will be a spasm end-feel. Allow time for relaxation of the muscle again. Hold–relax patterns can be used to maximize effectiveness. Slow, sustained stretches will produce the greatest gains.

LOWER TRAPEZIUS ACTIVATION

Biofeedback also can be used to enhance the activity of the lower trapezius during shoulder exercises. Often, the scapula will elevate during therapeutic exercises, which is not as effective as promoting scapular stability with humeral mobility (see figure 20.2).

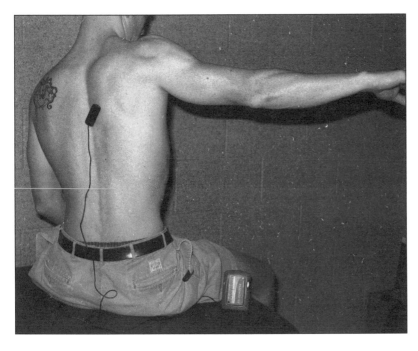

■ Figure 20.2 EMG biofeedback for lower trapezius. Electrodes are placed in parallel to the muscle fibers. The athlete should be able to see the unit and should try to activate the lower trapezius muscle during arm elevation.

Name_____ Date_____

Activities

1. To simulate the neuromuscular education that takes place with biofeedback, connect an EMG biofeedback device to the medial aspect of the first metatarsal on the belly of the adductor hallicus muscle. Have the volunteer attempt to adduct the toe. Adjust the threshold and gain so that minimal activity activates the EMG. When there is success, gradually increase the threshold so that a stronger contraction activates the EMG. Have some subjects try to learn how to raise an eyebrow with the same technique. Note your results here.

2. If two channels of an EMG are available, try to decrease activity in the vastus lateralis while increasing activity of the vastus medialis. This technique is used to promote medial tracking of the patella. Note your results here.

3. Use EMG biofeedback on the lower trapezius while performing shoulder abduction. The lower trap helps to stabilize the scapula in this manner. Note your results here.

CITED REFERENCES AND SUGGESTED READINGS

CITED REFERENCES

Currier DP: Neuromuscular stimulation for improving muscular strength and blood flow and influencing changes. In Nelson RM, Currier DP (Eds), *Clinical Electrotherapy*. Norwalk, CT, Appleton & Lange, 1991, 171-200.

Knight KL: *Cryotherapy: Theory, Technique and Physiology*. Chattanooga, TN, Chattanooga Corp., 1995.

Melzack R, Wall P: Pain mechanisms: A new theory. *Science* 150:971-979, 1965.

SUGGESTED READINGS

Alon G: Principles of electrical stimulation. In Nelson RM, Currier DP (Eds), *Clinical Electrotherapy*. Norwalk, CT, Appleton & Lange, 1991, 35-104.

Andersson GBJ, Schultz AB, Nachemson AL: Intervertebral disc pressures during traction. *Scand J Rehabil Med* 9:88-91, 1983.

Baker LL: Clinical uses of neuromuscular electrical stimulation. In Nelson RM, Currier DP (Eds), *Clinical Electrotherapy*. Norwalk, CT, Appleton & Lange, 1991, 143-170.

Baker LL: Neuromuscular electrical stimulation in the restoration of purposeful limb movements. In Wolf SL (Ed), *Electrotherapy: Clinics in Physical Therapy*. New York, Churchill Livingstone, 1981, 25-48.

Basmajian JV: The problem of the placebo in rehabilitation. *Physiother Can* 30:246-248, 1978.

Behnke RS: Cold therapy. *Athl Train, JNATA* 9:178-179, 1974.

Bender LF, Janes JM, Herrick JR: Histologic studies following exposure of bone to ultrasound. *Arch Phys Med Rehabil* 35:555-559, 1954.

Benson HAE, McElnay JC, Harland R: Phonophoresis of lignocaine and prilocaine from Emla cream. *Int J Pharm* 44:65-69, 1988.

Binder SA: Applications of low- and high-voltage electrotherapeutic currents. In Wolf SL (Ed), *Electrotherapy: Clinics in Physical Therapy*. New York, Churchill Livingstone, 1981, 1-24.

Bishop B: Pain: Its physiology and rationale for management. Part I: Neuroanatomical substrate of pain. *Phys Ther* 60:13-20, 1980.

Bishop B: Pain: Its physiology and rationale for management. Part II: Analgesic systems of the CNS. *Phys Ther* 60:21-23, 1980.

Bonica JJ: Anatomy and physiological basis of nociception and pain. In Bonica JJ (Ed), *The Management of Pain*. Philadephia, Lea & Febiger, 1990, 28-94.

Boone DC: Applications of iontophoresis. In Wolf SL (Ed), *Electrotherapy: Clinics in Physical Therapy*. New York, Churchill Livingstone, 1981, 99-122.

Borrell RM, Parker R, Henley EJ, Masley D, Repinecz M: Comparison of in vivo temperatures produced by hydrotherapy, paraffin wax treatment and fluidotherapy®. *Phys Ther* 60:1273-1276, 1980.

Brueton RN, Campbell B: The use of Geliperm as a sterile coupling agent for therapeutic ultrasound. *Physiotherapy* 73:653-654, 1987.

Buerskens AJ, vander Heijden GJ, de Vet HC, et al: The efficacy of traction for lumbar back pain: Design of randomized clinical trial. *J Manip Physiol Ther* 18:141-147, 1995.

Bugaj R: The cooling, analgesic, and rewarming effects of ice massage on localized skin. *Phys Ther* 55:11-19, 1975.

Byl NN: The use of ultrasound as an enhancer for transcutaneous drug delivery: Phonophoresis. *Phys Ther* 75:539-553, 1995.

Cameron MH, Monroe LG: Relative transmission of ultrasound by media customarily used for phonophoresis. *Phys Ther* 72:142-148, 1992.

Caolchis SC, Strohm BR: Cervical traction relationship of time to varied tractive force with constant angle of pull. *Arch Phys Med Rehabil* 46:815-819, 1965.

Carman KW, Knight KL: Habituation to cold-pain during repeated cryokinetic sessions. *J Athl Train* 27:223-228, 1992.

Castel JC: Therapeutic ultrasound. *Rehabil Ther Prod Rev* 22-31, Jan/Feb 1993.

Castel C, Draper DO, Castel D: Rate of temperature increase during ultrasound treatments: Are traditional treatment times long enough? *J Athl Train* 29:156-161, 1994.

Covington DB, Bassett FH: When cryotherapy injures. *Physician Sportsmed* 21:78-93, 1993.

Croce RV: The effects of EMG biofeedback on strength acquisition. *Biofeedback Self Regul* 11:299-306, 1986.

Cummings J: Iontophoresis. In Nelson RM, Currier DP (Eds), *Clinical Electrotherapy*. Norwalk, CT, Appleton & Lange, 1991, 317-330.

Cummings MS, Wilson VE, Bird EI: Flexibility development in sprinters using EMG biofeedback and relaxation training. *Biofeedback Self Regul* 9:295-301, 1984.

Currier DP, Greathouse D, Swift T: Sensory nerve conduction: Effect of ultrasound. *Arch Phys Med Rehabil* 59:181-185, 1978.

Deets D, Hands KL, Hopp SS: Cervical traction: A comparison of sitting and supine positions. *Phys Ther* 57:255-261, 1977.

Draper DO: A comparison of temperature rise in human calf muscle following applications of underwater and topical gel ultrasound. *J Orthop Sports Phys Ther* 17:247-251, 1993.

Draper DO, Hatheway C, Fowler D: Methods of applying underwater ultrasound: Science versus folklore. *J Athl Train* 26:83-87, 1991.

Draper DO, Sunderland S: Examination of the law of Grotthus-Draper: Does ultrasound penetrate subcutaneous fat in humans? *J Athl Train* 28:246-250, 1993.

Draper V: Electromyographic biofeedback and recovery of quadriceps femoris muscle function following anterior cruciate ligament reconstruction. *Phys Ther* 70:25-29, 1990.

Dyson M, Pond JB: The effect of pulsed ultrasound on tissue regeneration. *Physiotherapy* 56:136-142, 1970.

Dyson M, Sucking J: Stimulation of tissue repair by ultrasound: A survey of the mechanisms involved. *Physiotherapy* 64:105-108, 1978.

Farmer WC: Effect of intensity of ultrasound on conduction of motor axons. *Phys Ther* 42:1233-1237, 1968.

Gersh MR: Transcutaneous electrical nerve stimulation (TENS) for management of pain and sensory pathology. In Gersh MR (Ed), *Electrotherapy in Rehabilitation*. Philadelphia, Davis, 1992, 149-196.

Gieck JH, Saliba EN: Application of modalities in overuse syndromes. *Clin Sports Med* 6:427-466, 1987.

Goldish GD: A study of mechanical efficiency of split table traction. *Spine* 15:218-219, 1989.

Green GA, Zachazewski JE, Jordan SE: Peroneal nerve palsy induced by cryotherapy. *Physician Sportsmed* 17:63-70, 1989.

Griffin JE, Echternach JL, Price RE, Touchstone JC: Patients treated with ultrasonic driven hydrocortisone and ultrasound alone. *Phys Ther* 47:594-601, 1967.

Griffin JE, Karselis TC: *Physical Agents for Physical Therapists*. Springfield, IL, Charles C Thomas, 1982.

Hale JR, Jessen C, Fawcett AA, King RB: Arteriovenous anastomosis and capillary dilation and constriction induced by local heating. *Pflugers Arch* 404:203-207, 1985.

Halvorson G: Therapeutic heat and cold for athletic injuries. *Physician Sportsmed* 18:87-92, 1990.

Hanegan JL: Principles of nociception. In Gersh MR (Ed), *Electrotherapy in Rehabilitation*. Philadelphia, Davis, 1992, 26-47.

Hayes KB: *Manual for Physical Agents,* 4th ed. Norwalk, CT, Appleton & Lange, 1993, 1-2.

Ingersoll CD, Mangus BC: Habituation to the perception of the qualities of cold-induced pain. *J Athl Train* 27:218-220, 1992.

International Association for the Study of Pain: Pain terms: A list of definitions and notes on usage. *Pain* 14:205, 1982.

Isabell WK, Durrant E, Myrer W, Anderson S: The effects of ice massage, ice massage with exercise and exercise on the prevention and treatment of delayed onset muscle soreness. *J Athl Train* 27:208-217, 1992.

Kaempffe FA: Skin surface temperature reduction after cryotherapy to a casted extremity. *J Orthop Sports Phys Ther* 10:448-450, 1989.

Kahn J: *Low Volt Technique.* Syosset, NY, Joseph Kahn, 1983.

Kleinkort JA, Wood F: Phonophoresis with 1% versus 10% hydrocotisone. *Phys Ther* 55:1320-1325, 1975.

Knight K: The effects of hypothermia on inflammation and swelling. *Athl Train, JNATA* 8:7-10, 1976.

Knight KL: *Cryotherapy in Sport Injury Management.* Champaign, IL, Human Kinetics, 1995.

Kots YM: Electrostimulation. Paper presented at the Canadian-Soviet Exchange Symposium on Electrostimulation of Skeletal Muscles, Concordia University, Montreal, 1977.

LaBan MM, Macy JA, Meerschaert JR: Intermittent cervical traction: A progenitor of lumbar radicular pain. *Arch Phys Med Rehabil* 73:295-296, 1992.

Lehmann JF, DeLateur BJ, Silverman DR: Heating effects of ultrasound in human beings. *Arch Phys Med Rehabil* 47:331-339, 1966.

Lentell G, Hetherington T, Eagan J, Morgan M: The use of thermal agents to influence the effectiveness of a low-load prolonged stretch. *J Orthop Sports Phys Ther* 16:200-207, 1992.

Lota MJ, Darling RC: Change in permeability of the red blood cell membrane in a homogeneous ultrasonic field. *Arch Phys Med Rehabil* 36:282-286, 1955.

Maitland GD: *Vertebral Manipulation,* 5th ed. London, Butterworths, 1986.

Malone TR, Englehardt DL, Kirkpatrick JS, Bassett FH: Nerve injury in ahtletes caused by cryotherapy. *J Athl Train* 27:235-237, 1992.

Mannheimer JS, Lampe GN: *Clinical Transcutaneous Electrical Nerve Stimulation.* Philadelphia, Davis, 1984, 87-89.

McCulloch JM, Kemper CC: Vacuum therapy for the treatment of ischemic ulcer. *Phys Ther* 73:165-169, 1993.

McMaster WC: Cryotherapy. *Physician Sportsmed* 10:112-119, 1982.

Melzack R: Measurement of the dimensions of pain experience. In Bromm B (Ed), *Pain.* New York, Churchill Livingstone, 1987, 39-72.

Melzack R: The McGill Pain questionnaire. In Melzack R (Ed), *Pain Measurement and Assessment.* New York, Raven Press, 1983, 41-47.

Mersky H: Classification of chronic pain, descriptions of chronic pain syndromes and definition of pain terms. *Pain Suppl* 3:S10-S11, 1986.

Michlovitz SL: *Physical Agents.* Class notes, Hahnemann University, Broad and Vine Street, Philadelphia, 1988.

Michlovitz S, Firuta H: Peripheral edema: Pathophysiology, evaluation and management. *Postgrad Adv Phys Ther, APTA* 1987.

Miller CR, Webers RL: The effects of ice massage on an individual's pain tolerance level to electrical stimulation. *J Orthop Sports Phys Ther* 12:105-109, 1990.

Myer JW, Draper DO, Durrant E: Contrast therapy and intramuscular temperature in the human leg. *J Athl Train* 29:316-322, 1994.

Nanneman D: Thermal modalities: Heat and cold. *AAOHN J* 39:70-74, 1991.

Newton RA: Contemporary views on pain and the role played by thermal agents in managing pain symptoms. In Michlovitz SL (Ed), *Thermal Agents in Rehabilitation.* Philadelphia, Davis, 1990, 18-40.

Noonan TJ, Best TM, Anthony Seaber AV, Garrett WE: Thermal effects on skeletal muscle tensile behavior. *Am J Sports Med* 21: 517-522, 1993.

Olson JE, Stravino VD: A review of cryotherapy. *Phys Ther* 52:840-853, 1972.

Onel D, Tuzlaci M, Sari H, et al: Computed tomographic investigation of the effect of traction on lumbar disc herniations. *Spine* 14:82-90, 1989.

Patrick MK: Applications of therapeutic pulsed ultrasound. *Physiotherapy* 64:103-105, 1978.

Peek CJ: A primer of biofeedback instrumentation. In Schwartz MS (Ed), *Biofeedback: A Practitioner's Guide.* New York, Guilford Press, 1987, 87-106.

Pellecchia GL: Lumbar traction: A review of the literature. *J Orthop Sports Phys Ther* 20:262-267, 1994.

Price R, Lehmann JF, Boswell-Bessette S, Burleigh A, deLateur BJ: Influence of cryotherapy on spasticity at the human ankle. *Arch Phys Med Rehabil* 74:300-304, 1993.

Roberts M, Rutherford JH, Harris D: The effect of ultrasound on flexor tendon repairs in the rabbit. *Hand* 14:18-22, 1982.

Robinson SE, Buono MJ: Effect of continuous-wave ultrasound on blood flow in skeletal muscle. *Phys Ther* 75:145-150, 1995.

Rucinski TJ, Hooker DN, Prentice WE: The effects of intermittent compression on edema postacute ankle sprains. *J Orthop Sports Phys Ther* 14:65-69, 1991.

Saunders HD: Lumbar traction. *J Orthop Sports Phys Ther* 1:26-41, 1979.

Scudds RA: Pain assessment. *Aust J Physiol* 29:96-102, 1983.

Sloan JP, Giddings P, Hain R: Effects of cold and compression on edema. *Physician Sportsmed* 16:117-120, 1988.

Snyder-Mackler L: Electrical stimulation for pain modulation. In Snyder-Mackler L, Robinson AJ (Eds), *Clinical Electrophysiology*. Baltimore, Williams & Wilkins, 1989, 59-94.

Spielholz NI: Electrical stimulation of denervated muscle. In Nelson RM, Currier DP (Eds), *Clinical Electrotherapy*. Norwalk, CT, Appleton & Lange, 1991, 121-142.

Starkey C: *Therapeutic Modalities for Athletic Trainers*. Philadelphia, Davis, 1993, 1-22.

Stewart HF, Abjug JL: Contraindications in ultrasound therapy and equipment performance. *Phys Ther* 60:424-428, 1980.

Stratford PW, Levy DR, Gauldie S, Miseferi D, Levy K: The evaluation of phonophoresis and friction massage as treatments for extensor carpi radialis tendinitis: A randomized controlled trial. *Physiother Canada* 41:93-99, 1989.

Stratton SA: Role of endorphins in pain modulation. *J Orthop Sports Phys Ther* 3:200-205, 1982.

Strickler T, Malone T, Garrett W: The effects of passive warming on muscle injury. *Am J Sports Med* 18:141-145, 1990.

Twomey LT: Sustained lumbar traction: An experimental study of long spine segments. *Spine* 10:146-149, 1985.

Wilkerson GB: External compression for controlling traumatic edema. *Physician Sportsmed* 13:83-88, 1985.

Williams AR: *Ultrasound: Biological Effects and Potential Hazards*. London, Academic Press, 1983.

Williams AR, McHale J, Bowditch M, et al: Effects of ultrasound on electrical pain threshold perception in humans. *Ultrasound Med Biol* 13:249-251, 1987.

Yackzan L, Adams C, Francis K: The effects of ice massage on delayed onset muscle soreness. *Am J Sports Med* 12:159-165, 1984.

Ziskin MC, McDiarmid T, Michlovitz SL: Therapeutic ultrasound. In Michlovitz SL (Ed), *Thermal Agents in Rehabilitation*. Philadelphia, Davis, 1990, 134-169.

ABOUT THE AUTHORS

Susan Foreman Saliba, PhD, is a senior associate athletic trainer and a clinical instructor at the University of Virginia in Charlottesville, where she has taught therapeutic modalities for 12 years. A certified athletic trainer and licensed physical therapist, Dr. Saliba also taught therapeutic modalities at James Madison University in Harrisonburg, Virginia. She is chairperson of the National Athletic Trainers' Association Clinical Education Committee and a member of its Education Executive Committee. She earned a master's degree in athletic training and a PhD in sports medicine from the University of Virginia.

Ethan Saliba, PhD, has been teaching therapeutic modalities at the University of Virginia in Charlottesville for 18 years. He is currently head athletic trainer, overseeing 24 varsity sports. Dr. Saliba is a certified athletic trainer, licensed physical therapist, and sport certified specialist who has written extensively on various aspects of athletic injuries and rehabilitation. He earned a master's degree and PhD in sports medicine from the University of Virginia.

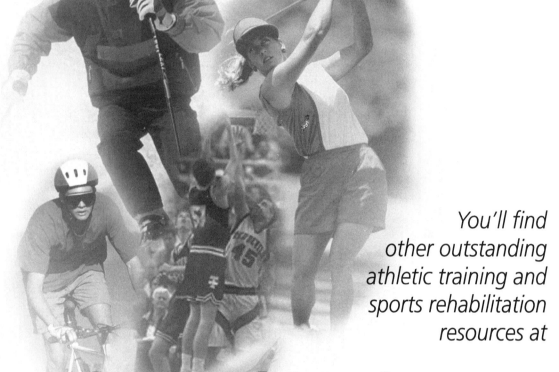

*You'll find
other outstanding
athletic training and
sports rehabilitation
resources at*

www.humankinetics.com

In the U.S. call

1-800-747-4457

Australia 08 8277 1555
Canada 1-800-465-7301
Europe .... +44 (0) 113 278 1708
New Zealand............................ 09-523-3462

HUMAN KINETICS
The Premier Publisher for Sports & Fitness
P.O. Box 5076 • Champaign, IL 61825-5076 USA